The Light in the Window

JUNE GOULDING

POOLBEG

Published 1998
by Poolbeg Press Ltd
123 Baldoyle Industrial Estate
Dublin 13, Ireland

© June Goulding 1998

The moral right of the author has been asserted.

A catalogue record for this book is available from the British Library.

ISBN 1 85371 892 0

Cover photography by Brigid Tiernan
Cover design by Poolbeg Group Services Ltd and Artmark
Set by Poolbeg Group Services Ltd in Stone 10/14.5
Printed by The Guernsey Press Ltd,
Vale, Guernsey, Channel Islands.

DEDICATION

To all those thousands of unmarried mothers and their babies who were incarcerated in that horrendous Home, especially those it was my privilege to nurse in 1951-52.

To Sister Hyacintha, who trained with me in 1950, and our friendship which was renewed many years later as the result of a coincidental meeting.

My special thanks to a schoolfriend from the Ursuline Convent in Sligo, who is a writer. She it was who typed the story from a pencil-written copybook. It could have ended up in the bin only for Mary Brennan Gaffney's encouragement.

A special word of thanks to my daughter Fiona, who keyed it into the computer, and who first joined the local creative writing class and got me to join soon afterwards. We were honoured to have Vincent McDonnell as our tutor. This book would never have been written without his guidance and enduring friendship. He gave me the confidence to send it off, and it is due to the enthusiasm and support of the late Kate Cruise O'Brien that it is now published.

My thanks to my dearest husband Pat for his love, patience, quiet help and consideration; to my sister Paddy in Manchester for all her letters and constant support; my seven children for their love and patience, and my love also to my thirteen grandchildren, who think I am cool!

Last but not least, my thanks to Sister Louis-Marie (O'Connor) who has been a constant friend. The saddest part of this dedication is that it was she who rang me in March of 1998 to tell me of Kate Cruise O'Brien's untimely death. I am at a loss to express my deep sadness, and may God comfort her husband Joe and son Alexander, and her friends and colleagues at Poolbeg Press.

To Kate: "Age cannot wither her, nor custom stale her infinite variety."
Shakespeare

Thank you, and God rest you.
June Goulding

CONTENTS

ONE

NO NIGHT DUTY

It was in August 1951, while I was working as a nurse on a private case, that my school-friend had her first baby. Full of excitement, I went to visit her in the maternity hospital where I had trained as a midwife up to the previous April. I smiled to myself as I wondered what it would have been like if she had given birth while I was on duty.

The weather was glorious – one of those hot days that we constantly remember from the summers of our youth – and the bright sunlight hurt my eyes after the continuous night duty. I was actually living in at the house where Séamus, a young man of twenty-four, was dying from tuberculosis of both lungs. He needed frequent morphine injections to calm him and help him to deal with the shortness of breath that squeezed the vibrancy from his body, and to offset any potential haemorrhaging. After some weeks of coming and going, it had been arranged that I sleep in an upstairs back bedroom, away from the traffic, so that I was "on call". I had had no day off, in all the twelve weeks that I nursed him.

A familiar feeling washed over me as I arrived at the hospital. I felt like walking briskly up the corridor and to the delivery room – it was difficult to credit that I was now simply another visitor bearing the customary bag of fruit and a knitted matinee coat. As I passed the Matron's office in the front hall I noticed that the door was ajar – probably for air circulation in the stifling conditions.

Catching my eye, the Assistant Matron called out: "You are the very one I want. How is your love life?" She had known that I was going out with a dental student during my training.

"Non-existent," I answered. "I'm on a private case since I left here last April."

"That's no place for you. Private nursing is very demanding and not very suitable for two lovebirds like you. Actually, a nun just rang a minute ago looking for a replacement for someone who's getting married. They want a nurse trained in this hospital and there's no night duty."

I found it hard to imagine a home or hospital without night duty. Half of my nursing career, which to date had included three years in general and one year in maternity, had been spent working the night shift.

"Where is this hospital?" I asked. "I don't believe a place that doesn't require night duty actually exists!"

"Before I give you details, would you consider going for an interview? Then, at least, you can judge for yourself," she insisted.

I agreed to this but stressed that I could not leave my patient as he had become very dependent on me. She then gave me the name and address of a home for unmarried mothers and directions on how to get there. I can truthfully say that I had no idea that such a place existed.

I left the office, clutching the piece of paper with the details, and trying to remain calm enough to concentrate on visiting the newly-delivered mother. By the time I had reached the ward and kissed her in congratulations, it was easier to forget that I had made a commitment to go for this interview. She proudly showed me her adorable daughter with her wrinkled features and wispy dark hair and went through the account of her labour. I had learnt that it was important for mothers to recount how they had come through this event and did my utmost to listen intently to her story.

Back out in the fresh air once more, I had time to think. I was certainly intrigued by the "no night duty" detail and remembered vividly how frantic the nights had been during my midwifery training. It was a case of just collapsing into bed as we came off duty only to begin the same thing on the following night. I paid the fare to the bus-conductor and grappled with thoughts of a job nursing unmarried mothers who had their babies in the daytime. In my naiveté, I thought that perhaps they might be different from other women. And I thought of Pat, my boyfriend, who was never able to meet me and take me for a drive or to a dance. I had no time off so we had to be content with communication by letters.

The next day, I wrote to him and told him of the job offer. Pat answered by return and said that he could never understand how my mother had allowed me to nurse an infectious tuberculosis patient as I had never contracted primary tuberculosis myself. He said that even though my lack of time off was upsetting him, he was far more concerned about the risk to my health. I hugged the letter close to my chest and thought that I was tired of conducting our relationship on paper – especially in view of the fact that we were engaged to be married.

The following week, I arranged the interview. Feeling disloyal for not disclosing my destination to my patient, I went home first to change and then set off on my bicycle on roads that knew nothing of the traffic that pounds on them today.

My heart was beating quickly, both from exertion and trepidation, as I slowed to negotiate the entrance to the Home. There were wrought-iron gates which hung on limestone pillars and as I went through I saw a tree-lined avenue. Everything seemed peaceful as I passed along by the well-trimmed shrubs and lawns. There was a lake to the right of the curving avenue and as I turned left I saw a square cement building surrounded by high walls with a small metal gate.

Propping my bicycle against the wall and carefully fixing my hair, I hoped that the effects of exertion were not too visible on my flushed cheeks. Taking a deep breath I pressed the bell on the side of the gate. Only the long row of upstairs windows, curtainless except for one, was visible from my vantage point.

A young girl, with dark circles under her eyes, took back a bolt and said: "Do you want Sister?" She was wearing some type of uniform and probably thought I was a prospective patient, as I had left my bicycle outside.

4

Closing and bolting the gate after I entered and bidding me to follow, she glanced quickly at me. My dress of red/white candy stripe, that had taken months to pay for at ten shillings a month, and my white sandals seemed so frivolous compared to her outfit I felt overdressed immediately.

I was led through a huge oak door that had a brass lock on the outside. Once in the hall, the girl went to a door marked *Office* and knocked. After what seemed an eternity to me, a white-clad nun emerged.

"Are you the nurse that was recommended from the maternity hospital?" she asked and looked me over with obvious disapproval. I regretted not wearing a costume that would fit these austere surroundings better but realised that my dress was far more suitable for the hot weather.

"Yes, Sister," I said. "I was asked by the Assistant Matron to come here for interview."

"We want a midwife," she corrected me pointedly and then turned to go into the office, gesturing me to follow. She was low-sized with steely grey eyes and a protruding lower jaw which gave her a determined expression. I swallowed hard, feeling at a disadvantage for the second time – I had not, as yet, become used to that title as I had only qualified sixteen weeks previously and spent twelve of those nursing Séamus.

The office seemed stark. It was small with a desk and chair and a glass panel that allowed full view of the long corridor that seemed to stretch forever over a shining parquet floor. She began to outline my duties and said that the position was live-in with a salary of eleven pounds, thirteen and fourpence which would be paid on the first day of every month.

"You will start on tomorrow week," she announced briskly.

"Sister," I interrupted and a brief expression of annoyance was visible on her face. "First I must tell you that I am on a private case – a young man of twenty-four who is dying of tuberculosis. I can hardly leave him now, especially when he has only weeks to live." My voice trailed off. She seemed unmoved, unconcerned.

"I want the position here filled by September 5th," she said.

"But Sister, Séamus may not die until the end of September. He's having terrible haemorrhages. Last week he had to have a blood transfusion after one severe haemoptasis." Again I faltered.

She stared at me.

"We need a midwife for September 5th. If you cannot start then, you are wasting my time."

Although it only took seconds, my mind seemed to spend forever churning up conflicting emotions. I could hear Pat saying "get out of that diseased atmosphere" and the assistant matron saying "no night duty – think of your love life". My own heart was torn between Séamus, who had become so dependent on me as his life was slowly coming to an end, and the prospect of working hours that left me with some time for living. If this were to happen today, I am sure I would have refused to be bullied into making my mind up. But in 1951 figures of authority – particularly those in religious life – were revered and obeyed as a matter of course.

I know now, with hindsight and forty-three years of regrets, that I was not strong enough to refuse to desert my patient in the last days of his life. I bitterly regret that

I left my post, nursing such a young man, for my own selfish reasons.

"All right, Sister," I said.

"Very well. I will take you on a tour of our hospital." It was like being back to my training days again as I followed her swishing skirt. I felt tired from the conflicting emotions and wished I could leave the whole scene. I remembered my boyfriend's suggestion that we go to England to get married and he could set up in private practice – this seemed like the ideal solution as I tried to quell the feeling that I would find it difficult to work with this stern woman.

The kitchens were opposite the office, with the usual noises of aluminium utensils clanging on stainless-steel draining-boards. I noticed the faint aroma of soup and baking as we passed along the spotless corridor.

Opening the first door on the left, I saw what I presumed was the girls' dining-room. White delph cups and saucers were set out on clothless timber tables. There were around ten or twelve tables with four straight-backed chairs around each. The door was opened into what she called the "dayroom". Forty or more blue-uniformed girls were sitting at a long table. There had been a babble of voices outside the door but, once the nun and I appeared, there was total silence and all heads were turned towards their knitting. A few looked up furtively.

"Get on with your knitting and no talking," the nun said in that tone that made me feel like a teenaged girl who had not learnt her algebra. Then we entered the labour ward. It contained two chromium beds and two chromium commodes, all of which were shining.

7

Pristine, crease-free sheets and covered pillows were on each bed. I noticed glass cases that contained instruments – needles and sutures – the usual equipment in a labour ward. A gleaming glass trolley which held a few stainless-steel bowls on the lower shelf stood along one wall. Everything, including the windows, walls and floors, was immaculately clean.

Outside this labour ward there was a small surgery with more glass cases and a sink. I noticed the urine-testing apparatus that explained the purpose of this room. The next door led into another room. I saw three-legged wooden stools stacked neatly along one wall. There were two large sinks and a canvas-topped table on folding legs. A few waste bins were here and there, and I saw a crucifix on the wall.

Then it was time to view the nursery. I was shown to a room which housed silver-painted metal cots in small and large sizes. There were babies in all the twelve or more cots. Two girls tended the infants who were whimpering, sleeping or crying. One of the girls put small Aspro-bottles with teats and what I presumed was sugar and water mixtures beside the mouths of the whimpering babies. The nun checked two or more of the babies and gave orders to the subservient girls who nodded but never spoke.

Finally I was shown to the ward where the newly-delivered girls slept with their babies in silver-painted metal carrycots beside them. There were eight beds here and four were divided by glass partitions. Again, gleaming chromium seemed to be everywhere. Cotton sheets and white spreads covered the beds. There were four or five girls in this ward – most of whom were breastfeeding their infants.

"Now I will show you your flat," I was told as if I were being led to a suite in the Dorchester! I followed her up the white marble staircase and along another polished corridor. My dining-room was first. Here muslin curtains framed the windows – I remembered seeing them on my arrival at the formidable cement high wall that encircled the hospital. This room was furnished with oak chairs and a table.

An electric fire was housed in a mock fireplace. Hanging on the wall, over the shelf that acted as a mantelpiece, was a cross bearing the crucified figure of Christ. A wireless stood on a shelf near the armchair. The walls were painted in gloss paint in a cream colour. The parquet floor was highly polished and the curtains did not obliterate the magnificent view of the lake and rolling lawns that reached down through a myriad of shrubs.

Sister said: "Your bathroom is across the corridor and next to the dining-room is your bedroom."

This contained a three-and-a-half-foot bed with a white candlewick bedspread. There was a wardrobe and a tallboy and dressing-table. A porcelain hand-basin gleamed from its corner position. Behind the bed there was a hatch which drew my attention but I did not want to ask any questions. By now I was not sure of my plans. I could not help thinking that I was deserting Séamus, but the thought of a spotless flat of my own with no night duty certainly appealed to me.

"Next door to your room is a twenty-bed dormitory where the girls nearest their due dates sleep," she announced suddenly.

We descended the stairs in silence and I followed her into the office once more.

"I'll need to know in forty-eight hours if you are accepting the position. Good day."

I was shown to the main door and curtly dismissed. This was my introduction to the woman who held power over three hundred and fifty unfortunate girls in a secret penitential jail. I have chosen to call her simply "Sister" in this book. Those who knew her will remember her.

The warmth of the sun acted like a balm to my senses as I searched for my bicycle. The interview had been an intimidating experience but then there were no courses on interviewing skills in 1951. Once I had come to terms with my decision, I was left with the terrible dread of giving my notice.

Pedalling with a strength born from anxiety, I soon arrived back home, just in time for tea. It was difficult to recount the afternoon in detail as my parents and siblings clamoured for information.

As we ate slices of sponge cake and drank tea they tried to make me feel better about leaving Séamus prematurely and planned how I could spend some of my off-duty at home. One glance at the clock and it was time to set off on my bicycle once more. Each yard made me feel more the traitor.

"Good, he's been calling for you," Séamus' aunt said on my return. Before I had time to tell her of my decision I could hear my name being faintly called by Séamus.

While I was preparing to give him his shot, he caught my hand and said that we would go to visit the Burren, West Cork and Kerry when he was better. The euphoria, that seized him at times and which was common to tuberculosis patients, was heartbreaking, but even more so when I held my secret deep in my heart. Soon he was sleeping and I longed to rush from his room and tell that nun that I would not be able to start until my work here was finished. However, fear that this would jeopardise the whole turnabout in my career and fear at being treated harshly for breaking my agreement with her invaded my soul and I sat, torn with guilt, and watched the shallow breathing of the man I soon would abandon.

"You can't be serious – he depends so much on you," his aunt said, later as she stirred her tea round and round.

"I'm so sorry. If there was any other way – I hope you'll understand that this job is incredibly difficult on my fiancé and me as we have had little or no time together for the past twelve weeks. I tried to explain to my prospective employer but she needed to fill the position immediately."

It was hopeless. The words sounded wrong and I knew that I was causing great pain in this woman who doted on her nephew.

"You'll have to tell him yourself," she said finally in a quiet voice as she held her hand over her mouth as if to steady herself.

The hours ticked slowly by that week but each time that I tried to broach the subject, Séamus made plans for what we would do when he improved or else was simply too weak to be burdened with further problems. With only two days to go, I got up slowly and wearily from a disturbed night's sleep and told myself that my health would not have taken much more of this job in any case. As I approached his room, his aunt suddenly appeared and shook her head from side to side. I knew that she had told him and paused before I entered the room.

"Séamus," I began. He looked at me. One long stare from those frightened eyes and then he turned his head to the wall. I tried to explain but for the final hours of my duty with him he refused to acknowledge my presence – as if it was the last piece of dignity afforded to him. My time there humbled me greatly but I comforted myself in the knowledge that there were better things ahead. How foolish could I have been?

TWO

LEAVING SÉAMUS

It was September 5th. My eyes were blinded by tears as I walked towards my fiancé's waiting car. The two cases that held my belongings seemed light in comparison with the heavy burden in my heart. Séamus had been sleeping after that final injection when I slipped out of the house.

"Give me those – thank God you are out of there – do you ever think of yourself or me?" Pat said as he held me close.

I was too upset to talk much during the journey to my new job.

"What are your off-duty hours here, or are you once more going to be inaccessible?" he said suddenly.

"Oh! Shut up! It's no picnic for me either. Do you think I enjoy not being able to meet you?"

We laughed then, realising the foolishness of picking on each other in our few minutes together. I asked him to drop me at the main gate despite his insistence that the cases were quite heavy. I needed time to be alone before I entered that building. Promising to write with immediate news of my next day off, we kissed and held each other briefly before I got out of the car.

The walk gave me time to calm myself with thoughts. I had been told that there were 350 girls staying at this place and the thought of all those deliveries frightened me. As I approached the hospital I could see the convent nearby. It was a large, ivy-covered Georgian house, facing south and overlooking the lake. As I admired the immaculate lawns and driveway I wondered who maintained them in such excellent condition as I could not see any team of gardeners or men pausing to mop sweat from their brows with well-worn caps.

The green lawns were edged with shrubs – rhododendrons, lilac and spirea – which no doubt would stand dark and forbidding during the winter months, but were a riot of colour today. I heard the murmur of bees, attracted by the bounty of flowers, and heard the birds singing as if over-burdened with joy at being alive on such a day. My heart lifted – it was going to be all right. Perhaps nature was telling me that I had made the right decision.

When I had knocked at the big oak door once more, the nun who had interviewed me and who obviously was in charge bade me enter. My two cases seemed so ridiculous under her gaze but I declined to tell her that I was working on my trousseau. Somehow I felt that she would not understand the comfort of hand-stitching silk underwear and nightdresses.

She called a girl to show me to my room, managed to

14

arrange her features into a smile, and said: "You will need to come down to the nursery at five o'clock for the bathing and feeding of the babies."

I followed the girl, who had insisted on carrying my cases up the stairs. She never spoke and I wondered if she missed the previous nurse and resented my arrival.

"What's your name?" I asked once we had arrived at my room.

She stopped and stared at me and then glanced furtively over her shoulder.

"It's Irene. It's not my real name, Nurse, but anyway we're not supposed to talk."

I was amazed. Was I to be given the silent treatment in order that I know my place, I wondered? Slowly walking over to close my door I explained that she could whisper if it made her feel any better.

She told me that she was from Kerry and had a little boy, Seán, aged three, who was over at the main convent. She then explained that she would be serving me meals in this room and was responsible for any jobs I needed doing. I felt embarrassed at having a "girl Friday" but realised that she seemed to take pride in this position.

Once she had left, I hung up my clothes, and put some face-cloths by the hand-basin along with a bar of lily-of-the-valley soap that my sisters had given me as a good luck present. I changed into my nurse's uniform and went into the little sitting-room as I had a few minutes to spare. The view was spectacular and peaceful but my thoughts flew back to Séamus. I remembered Pat's words: "All that morphine will dull his senses – don't worry too much." I looked up at the crucifix, said a silent prayer and prepared to go to work.

I reported at the office, where Sister was waiting for me. She appeared pleased at my uniform and the fact that I was punctual but said nothing.

"First we will go to the newly-delivered mothers' ward. We allow them to stay in bed for ten days after their babies are born," she said briskly and her veil swung from side to side as she walked. She said these women stayed in the Home after the birth and worked there until their babies were three years old. The children were then fostered and the mothers were free to go.

The information registered in my brain as I tried to keep up with her rhythmic footsteps. I could not imagine why the babies were not placed in care immediately after the birth to avoid trauma on both sides. Wanting to query the soundness of this procedure, I bit my lip and decided to wait until I had become more accustomed to the practices of the hospital before questioning their wisdom.

At the door of the ward she paused and outlined some of the rules and conditions pertaining to my position. I soon learnt that the hatch behind my bed opened directly into the dormitory of the girls who were near their due dates.

"If any girl goes into labour in the night they will knock on the hatch for you," she said.

"I thought that there was no night duty?" I said as a sinking feeling washed over me.

"Well," she said, "I sleep in the convent so you are in charge of the deliveries at night – if there are any." She then walked swiftly through the door and I had no time to deal with the sense of anxiety that pervaded my thoughts.

Four newly-delivered mothers with their babies sleeping peacefully in their cots were in the ward.

Directly to the right of the door I saw a red-haired girl attempting to breast-feed a tiny infant while holding a swab of cotton wool to a suppurating abscess. The fact that she would have needed three hands to successfully complete this task was a minor obstacle when compared to the obvious agony on her face. Tears ran unchecked down her pale face and she did not look up to acknowledge our presence.

"Don't let the pus into the baby's mouth," commanded Sister curtly as she walked to another bed.

I was dumbfounded. It was quite obvious that each time the hungry baby gulped its mother's milk the pain in her infected breast became excruciating. I had previously nursed unfortunate women in the training hospital with blocked milk ducts whose temperatures shot up to 103 degrees. We tried to ease their acute discomfort with hot face-cloths and four-hourly dosages of aspirin. When this did not arrest the problem they were put on penicillin. I had never before seen an abscess that had actually created such an enormous open wound.

"Sister," I whispered in muted tones in an effort to avoid alarming the distressed patient. "Is she on antibiotics?"

The reply came as a withering look as the nun continued to glance at the other mothers and order them to give the babies ten minutes at each breast. My heart pounded as I followed her. What could I do now? Could it be possible that this girl had to suffer without medical intervention? Was this the case, or did the Sister mean that I was stating the obvious by suggesting antibiotics? I was overwhelmed by a sense that the atmosphere was almost penitential but tried to tell myself that I was full of first-day nerves and probably over-reacting.

After that initiation, I was led to the nursery where sixteen young girls were sitting in a semicircle on milking stools. Each held a baby aged from six weeks to nine months and I was told that I would be responsible for the undressing and bathing of these babies. They should then be handed back to their mothers for breast-feeding.

I watched as she supervised the feeding process and I felt that her attitude would have been more fitting at an army barracks. She handed one girl's newborn infant to a mother with a three-months-old baby who was being breast-fed every four hours. I waited for an outcry or a complaint from each of the mothers but noticed that they hung their heads and tried to bite their trembling lips. Memories of an incident in the training hospital when a young trainee had inadvertently brought the wrong baby to be fed came to my mind. The mother who had failed to discover the mistake until after feeding the infant could not be consoled. The violation of this natural maternal instinct seemed to be common practice in this Home and I found it difficult to breathe evenly as I witnessed it.

I was intimidated into a silence that I found crushing as it was obvious that Sister had ultimate control over each and every sphere of this hospital. I longed to storm out, hand in my notice and run away. I felt trapped but knew that if I balked at my responsibilities at this early stage I would probably never secure another position. The tension emanating in the room made me realise that confrontation with this figure of authority would probably create more problems than it would solve.

Trying to concentrate solely on bathing the babies and supervising the feeding, I promised myself to do the thinking later. When this job was finished and the babies settled into their cots for the night, the girls returned, I was told, to the dayroom. I reported back to the Sister's office as I had been instructed.

Before being dismissed for the night she outlined some more rules. I was not allowed any contact with the girls except in a professional manner. I was only permitted to talk to them in relation to the date of their babies' arrivals.

"You are not to get familiar with any of the girls and you most certainly will never post a letter for them. Is that quite clear, Nurse Goulding?"

I nodded, upset by the expression on her face and wearily went up to my quarters. It was half-nine, and I wondered if I could get used to being institutionalised in this place. My flat seemed tarnished by the sensation that I would be expected to adhere to rules that seemed to me grossly unfair. As I washed, and put on my night clothes, I thought of Pat, of home and of Séamus and felt a familiar lump rise in my throat.

Once in bed I pulled myself up to a sitting position and opened the hatch quietly. There were two girls settled in the twenty-bedroomed dormitory.

"Are you the new nurse?" one said tentatively. "We heard a new nurse would be coming."

They explained that they were in bed early as their babies were due and they had been instructed to knock on the hatch if the pains came during the night. The

19

other girls sharing the dormitory would be up at around ten but would make no noise, they said. I noticed their guarded expressions and told them that they could knock on the hatch at any time. We said goodnight to each other and as I shut the hatch it became clear to me why I was to have no regular night duty.

Like a GP, I was obviously on call twenty-four hours a day. My day duty hours were from half-eight in the morning to eight at night. I would be expected to cope with night deliveries and be on duty the following day also. And to think that I had taken this job to ensure that I would have more time off!

The other facts that the nun had make known to me also filled me with anxiety. It came as a shock to discover that she was the only nun in the Home who was a qualified midwife. The fact that this was the case would have been quite common at that time as, prior to 1950, religious sisters were the protected species and were not allowed to train in midwifery. During the reign of Pope Pius XII this rule was changed. I wondered how this nun and I could cope with delivering all those babies without back-up.

THREE

FIRST OFFENDERS

It was no use. Sleep refused to come. As it was not yet ten o'clock, I slipped on a dressing-gown and went downstairs to see if I could make myself a cup of coffee and, perhaps, to meet someone who would enlighten me further about this home for unmarried mothers.

Directly under my bedroom was the night nursery for the new babies. The dim light could be seen from the bottom of the stairs so I crept along the corridor. As I tried to open the door of the nursery, a tall woman of about fifty opened it and said: "Good night. Are you the new nurse? Sister told us that you were arriving tonight."

Once I had explained who I was and where I was going, I took time to notice the sixteen wooden cots lined in white calico once more. A young girl of about nineteen was helping to soothe the fretful babies. I was told that she helped the night attendant but that she had a nine-month-old baby girl herself.

21

Walking around the cots, I could not help but admire these babies. All the infants in the maternity hospital where I had trained had barely changed from the very new baby stage when they left with their proud parents. These older babies, two to four months, with their fair, dark or red hair were the most beautiful group of babies I had ever seen.

"Would you like to come to the kitchen, as I make tea at this time every night?" the tall woman asked.

"I'd love a cup of coffee but most of all I'd like to find out more about this place," I replied.

Soon we were sitting by the Aga in the spacious kitchen and I enjoyed a cup of coffee with some hot buttered toast. The night attendant, Colette, told me that the previous nurse had left to get married after seven years in the Home. She seemed reluctant to offer information and answered my questions in monosyllables. I was relieved to learn that there were only forty girls in the hospital – twenty of whom were heavily pregnant. Those who had their babies went to live in the convent where they would rear their children until they would be fostered at the age of three.

Back in my room once more, taking off my dressing-gown, I looked at the hatch and silently prayed that there would not be any early call. Frankly, I was scared as I knew that I was all alone and there would be no doctors to be called in a crisis.

Sleep almost escaped me on that first night. Towards dawn I drifted into a heavy sleep to be awakened again by the soft footsteps of the girls in the adjoining dormitory. I peeped out and watched them sleepily and wearily make their way down the oak corridor and down the stairs to put on their shoes. I had noticed the tidy heap under the marble staircase on the previous night.

"Where are you going?" I asked one of the girls.

"To Mass, Nurse," she said.

"Why do you leave your shoes downstairs – is it to avoid making noise?"

"No, Nurse – Sister said we might mark the steps," came the reply.

I returned to my room and splashed my face with cold water. I had considered going to Mass but now felt too cross and confused after this snippet of information. I wanted to rail at the woman who thought the risk of dirtying a staircase outshone the risk of bulky-framed pregnant girls slipping in their stockinged feet.

Once I had washed and dressed, I made my bed and wondered what to do next. A tentative knock at the door followed and Irene came in with a tray. My breakfast consisted of cornflakes, bacon and egg, bread and tea. She laid it gently on the table in the dining-room and smiled at me.

"Thank you, Irene," I said and noticed her blush as she left the room.

I felt guilty at savouring the meal in the privacy of my own flat whilst the inmates had to walk barefoot from their beds. Once I had finished, I checked that my hair was tidily pinned up beneath my veil, smoothed the few crumbs from my uniform and set about returning my tray to the kitchen.

On my way there, I met Irene who took the tray from me and said:

"You mustn't do that. It's my job to look after you, Nurse – I'm sorry for not coming up sooner."

Once again I thanked her and made my way to the day nursery. There were twelve babies to be bathed that day. My confidence came back to me as I tightly wound a towel around a squirming baby and held his dark head over the sink. I washed his face and hair first and then, removing the towel, cradled him in the crook of my arm as I slowly lowered him in the warm water. As usual his hands clenched and his arms flew out in reflex action. It was comforting to know that babies were babies at bath time no matter what the circumstances!

Once the task had been completed, I wrapped him in a towel and handed him to his mother to dry and dress.

"Don't forget the creases under his chin – pat them gently," I said and noticed that his mother tenderly dried his wet glistening body as if he were made of the finest porcelain.

This room had two sinks and a few canvas-topped tables for dressing the babies. It was facing south so the morning sun poured in through the French doors that opened on to a well-trimmed lawn. As the babies were bathed and dressed the mothers sat on the wooden stools to feed them.

Sister duly arrived in her white habit with a large crucifix of silver on her flattened chest. She supervised the bathing and feeding in her tight-lipped manner. Again this was all new to me as there were some babies as old as ten and twelve months still being breast-fed by very tired and transparent-looking mothers.

At eleven, I was instructed to examine those girls nearest their delivery dates. I followed her to the dayroom.

"All the girls in here are first offenders and they are

very lucky to have such a place to come," was her remark as she called about four or five girls and told them to go to the labour ward to be examined. With that she walked off to the convent. There was an immediate sense of relief that was palpable.

One girl followed me silently to the appointed room and the others waited silently in the small adjacent surgery. There was a small wooden stool beside the bed in the labour ward so that they could climb up more easily. Slowly the very heavily pregnant girl approached.

"I'm overdue," she said. God love her, she was but seventeen, with long black hair tied back in a rubber band. Her shapeless blue smock hung limply over the huge "bump". Soon the tension was easing as she started to talk.

"We're all glad you came. Sister was alone here since the other nurse left. We all have different names here, but Sister says we are all the same and it was the same thing that landed us in here. We have to stay here for three years and then part with our babies."

It began to dawn on me that this place was more like a penitentiary than a nursing home. My work with these unfortunate "fallen women" would be an eye-opener to a different part of life of which I had been previously unaware. I took her blood pressure and recorded it. I tested the sample of urine. Taking out my foetal stethoscope, I helped her to push the dress up over her abdomen. Once I had listened to and recorded the foetal heartbeat and palpated for any unusual presentation, I noticed the coarse material of her knickers. They were made of a blue denim-like fabric with a drawstring on top and looked like the present-day boxer shorts. I was about to comment that they looked very uncomfortable when I realised that this comment would be of no help to the girl whatsoever.

"I notice that you are not wearing a bra – are your breasts sore or something?" I asked.

She shifted uncomfortably and I helped her to a sitting position and readjusted her clothing.

"We're not allowed, Nurse – this is our uniform and these are the knickers. The girls who are feeding their babies say that it feels much worse on their chests then without support."

"I see," was all I could think of saying. Would I cause more discomfort by telling those girls that I thought that the rules were appalling? Was there any point in tackling the nun about the importance of comfortable underwear during pregnancy? I sensed that my advice would go unheeded.

The next girl that I examined was well beyond her due date and I had been instructed to shave her pubic hair in preparation for the birth. I noticed how sore she looked as I tried to be gentle – how I longed to get a big jar of Vaseline to smear on her red raw groins. She was most uncomplaining and it was obvious that she was not used to normal conversation in this place.

It was quiet that day – no baby decided to arrive. I had time to work with the babies and the mothers and time to adapt to my new surroundings. I sat in the dayroom for a while, listening to the clicking of knitting-needles as the girls knitted matinee coats for their expected babies.

I wondered how I would manage on my first delivery and yet felt glad that I had a little time to get used to this place. As I lay in bed that night I heard the sound of muffled sobs from the dormitory. On opening the hatch I asked if the girl in question was all right.

"She cries herself to sleep every night, Nurse," came the reply.

* * *

It was about five-thirty on a late September morning when the hatch above my iron bed was abruptly knocked upon and then shoved in. A girl's worried face appeared at the opening.

"Nurse," she whispered. "One of the girls is getting the pains but the waters have just broken."

I put on my dressing-gown and went into the dormitory. Most of the girls were propped up on one elbow and all were scared, half sleepy and trying to find out what was happening. Some were crying. None slept. They knew very little of the details of the actual birth, as I was to find out later. The young girl who was helping the night attendant was trying to help the girl in labour out of the bed.

"Nurse," she said. "I wet the bed – Sister will be going mad."

"It's not your fault," I said. "Your waters have broken. You will have your baby today. Don't worry. I will get dressed and be back to take you down to the labour ward. It will be all right."

One of the girls in an adjoining bed said: "Don't worry, Nurse. We will wash her sheet and Sister will never know."

In the grey light of dawn, all their faces looked ghost-like. So this was my first delivery in the Home. I was less than a week in residence. I was scared. The story of the wet sheet was the first indication for me of the fear that Sister had instilled. Childbirth was not fear enough.

Hurriedly I put on my uniform and went to the dimly-lit ward. I found the girl in an advanced state of labour and as she looked at me pleadingly I held her hand in an effort to reassure her. After examining her I enquired what analgesic was available. I was unprepared for Colette's embarrassment as she walked to the sink and said: "Nobody gets anything here, Nurse. They just have to suffer."

Jesus, I thought, what in God's name brought me to such a place? I remembered my training days in the maternity hospital and the "twilight sleep" that had been in vogue since 1948 when the then Princess Elizabeth gave birth to Prince Charles. How very far removed was this place of torture from the training hospital and even more distanced from Buckingham Palace!

Shortly after nine, Sister swished along the oak corridor and arrived at the Nursery to carry out the bathing routine. She was after eight o'clock Mass and Holy Communion and, no doubt, a good breakfast over with her Community in the convent.

I transferred the girl in labour into a white calico gown and put her onto the labour-ward bed. I did not know whether to stay with her as her contractions were coming strong every two minutes. (We were never allowed leave a patient in labour alone in the maternity hospital where I trained). I wondered if I should start the daily routine of bathing the babies before the ten o'clock feed. I was not left long in the dark.

Sister took a look at the girl in labour and made her get

up and sit on one of the chromium commodes. She asked me to put a blanket around her shoulders and said: "Now we start the bathing in the nursery."

I got a small wooden stool for the young girl's legs and whispered a word of encouragement in her ear as I pulled the blanket more firmly around her shoulders. "I'll be back as soon as I can to you," I said in as low a voice as I could.

The waiting patients carried on with their daily chores of polishing and cleaning and high dusting and whatever it was that kept all forty of the nearest to their delivery dates so busy in the morning. This particular day, there were no girls examined in the labour ward as was the usual practice, on account of the girl in labour.

Sister came in and checked on her progress by making her bend over. It was possible to see if there was any pressure on her anal area in the highly polished chromium commode. Tentatively, I suggested letting the girl back up on the bed.

Sister said: "No, she is not ready yet." I was hoping that she would go over to the convent – this was the first birth that I was to attend and I really was not sure of my position or my duties in the labour ward. The poor girl was nearing the end of her labour and was admonished several times for moaning out loud. This, or any attempt at screaming, was forbidden and a smart lecture ensued.

I asked Sister to allow the girl back on the bed so that I could check the foetal heartbeat. Sitting on a commode was neither comfortable or conducive to proper monitoring of the foetal heartbeat. In the next half-hour, I was able to deliver the baby while Sister grudgingly allowed me to put the girl on her left side on the bed.

After I tied the umbilical cord and placed the new baby boy in a towel to weigh him, I then delivered the afterbirth and eventually gave the infant to his mother. Like every newly-delivered mother I had attended to, she kissed and hugged and admired her son while I tried to make her comfortable as Sister walked over to her lunch in the convent.

There was no fuss. No girl was allowed into the labour ward to see the new arrival – it was a non-event. Later in the early afternoon, the girl had to walk down the corridor to the ward where there were three newly-delivered mothers.

I was relieved and excited that all went well. I could not help thinking of the deliveries in the maternity hospital where I had trained, with the gynaecologist, the house surgeon, the labour ward sister, two staff nurses, about three student nurses and three medical students. It was like a team, with the gas and oxygen and pethedine at hand.

I wondered if "no night duty" was too high a price to pay. It is only now, with hindsight, that I suppose my youth was on my side as I had little else going for me.

That night I went down to visit my first new baby and mother several times. Colette came on again at nine. and we chatted once more over tea and toast by the Aga. She told me that she had come from Wexford. She had had a son thirty years previously and remained on after he was fostered. She never knew where he had been placed. As her family disowned her, she opted to remain on in the Home as night attendant. To my knowledge, she never got a salary or a night off in twenty-five years.

As we chatted, I felt safe to ask her about something that had been bothering me all day.

"Colette," I said, almost in whisper. "When I delivered that girl today, I went to the glass cabinet for some sutures – after all, her son was almost nine pounds in weight and she was so young. She had a slight tear and I felt it would be wise to insert one stitch. Sister refused to give me the key and insisted that there was absolutely no need to stitch her." I faltered, feeling embarrassed and ashamed at not standing my ground. I wanted to tell Colette that I found it impossible to do my duties as midwife when the Sister had such a domineering attitude in the labour ward.

Colette shook her head from side to side and chased stray crumbs on the plate with her index finger.

"I'm afraid, Nurse, the key to that cabinet has never been handed over. Girls must suffer their pain and put up with the discomfort of being torn – she says that they should atone for their sin."

I got up abruptly from the table muttering something about being tired. I walked quickly towards the convent, determined to tell the Sister that I would no longer be available to work in such a harsh regime. I wanted to scream at her that I was trained to make pregnant women as comfortable as possible during the delivery and afterwards, and that, apart from my horror at the cruelty I was witnessing, the rules in this place were making a mockery of my training.

"Nurse," I heard Colette call softly after me. I waited as she caught up. "One of the girls has started upstairs." She looked at my face, as if knowing my thoughts. "Where were you going?" she asked.

31

"Nowhere," I said as I followed her upstairs to the labour ward. As I prepared to deliver another baby, I made my mind up to try and show as much kindness as I could to these pathetic girls without creating problems with Sister. I knew, deep in my heart, that she would have the power to fire me and perhaps hire somebody more willing to treat these girls as criminals.

"I'm glad you came, Nurse," said Colette as we helped the young girl into her gown. I wished I could echo her sentiment.

FOUR

GIVING UP ASSUMPTA

I awoke early the following morning. Instead of going to Mass, I went to the newly-delivered mothers' ward. I found a trolley on which I put bowls of Dettol, swabs and bedpans.

My little mother of the day before was vainly trying to breast-feed her son with advice coming from the competent mothers all around her – all of whom were under twenty years old! The other girl that had been delivered early in the morning lay in her bed, shattered, staring at the ceiling. The memories of her excruciating labour had obviously not dimmed since I had settled her at two o'clock in the morning. Her eight-pound daughter whimpered softly in the nearby cot.

Deciding to leave her alone for a while, I put each mother in turn on the warmed stainless-steel bedpan and then, after they had passed urine, I swabbed them and put on a fresh pad. These pads consisted of wads of cotton wool encased in gauze. When it was quiet in the labour ward, I used to make them as I had been trained in the hospital. The condition of the girls' bruised and torn perineums bore no relation to those of the women I had swabbed in the training hospital. Though they must have been feeling very sore, they smiled gratefully at me as I tried to be gentle.

I then went over to my first-born delivery and helped his mother to breast-feed him. Once he was latched on successfully, I looked at the next cubicle. To my surprise the little girl was feeding contentedly at her exhausted mother's breast.

"Good girl, Anne, I was going to give her a bottle of glucose and water to give you a chance. You'd a tough time, God help you."

"Thanks, Nurse," she said, almost in tears. "I thought I might as well try and feed her – it wasn't her fault that I'm in here."

I wondered, silently, where the child's father was at this moment. When I had finished, I returned to my flat where Irene had left my breakfast tray. On her return, we talked briefly – she always had one eye on the door and was terrified of being caught talking to me. She told me that word had gone round that I was different from the former nurse and that I was "all for the patients".

"That's what I am paid for here, Irene. I am the new midwife. I will deliver all the girls that I can."

"Nurse," she said, "all the waiting girls are hoping that they can hold on for you. Sister leaves them too long on the commode."

"Don't worry. Colette and I will work something out."

"Nurse, Sister told me that I was to do your laundry as well as your meals.

"Just my uniform so, I'll do my own undies, but thank you all the same," I said, embarrassed at this service. "Tell me," I asked. "How long are you here?"

"Three years, Nurse," she said. "I have a son of three over in the convent. He is soon going." Her eyes filled up with tears as she took my tray. "It's great you are here – we all feel we have one friend now."

"I can do very little for you, Irene," I said. "I wish I could do more but the rules are so rigid and Sister seems in complete command."

As she left my room it was becoming more and more apparent to me that this place of detention was more like a prison than a home.

I was becoming more accustomed to the routine and tried to enjoy the tension-free moments when Sister was not looking over my shoulder. Most mornings at about eleven o'clock, Reverend Mother Rosamund came over from the convent to do her rounds of the hospital. She was a fat jolly woman with a ready smile for everyone – very different from the white-clad Sister in charge of the hospital.

There were usually around forty waiting girls and twenty newly-delivered mothers in the hospital. When the babies were three to four months old they and their mothers were sent over to the convent, where about three hundred girls and their children of one, two or three years lived with the community of nuns.

The Bessboro Estate was originally owned in the 17th century by the Pike family who were Quakers. There were eventually two unmarried sisters who died without issue.

A man from Langford Row bought the Estate for a nominal sum and then sold it to the English Order of The Sacred Heart of Jesus and Mary. The Order also owned and ran the Castlepollard Home for unmarried mothers, Co Westmeath. Mostly Irish women entered this order.

I began to learn more about the rules of the Home, like the fact that the Cork Corporation Rates paid £1.00 for each girl and 2/6d for each baby, per week, to the convent. Each girl had to stay and work for three years to help with the running of the Home and self-supporting farm. During this time their babies were breastfed for 12 months after which they were fed on goody (bread soaked in milk) and creamed potatoes every day. On Sunday mornings, the girls were given sausages (these were boiled in roasting tins in the Aga) for their breakfast. Every one of the convent girls carefully hid those sausages in their smock pockets and fed them later to their growing babies. That meant that these young mothers had bread and margarine seven days a week for breakfast and tea. They got two boiled eggs in a week for tea.

After the three years the babies were sent out to foster homes or orphanages or else adopted. The mothers were allowed to go free with little or no money and only the clothes they came in with. Few if any went home to their parents, having left the parish to avoid bringing disgrace on the family, they were no longer welcome back.

Only a small minority of girls whose family could pay £100 (a fortune in 1951) to the nuns, were free to leave ten days after the birth of their baby. Their babies were immediately available for adoption. It was usually the girls' mothers that brought them in to the Home and took care of this transaction. Having a baby out of wedlock was such a taboo subject at the time that often these women did not even tell their husbands that their daughter was pregnant. Instead they consulted the parish priest who usually advised that the girl would be better off going to one of these homes, away from the locality.

There was one other way of escape without the baby. If a girl's family had £50, her baby would be sent out to a foster home in the city and then, after ten days, the girl would be free to go. No girl could keep her baby or go home with her baby no matter what her family paid.

* * *

Three weeks after starting work I decided that I should call to see Séamus when I came off duty one evening. I cycled up to his aunt's house, about five miles from the Home. I was apprehensive at the thought of meeting him again. I was shown in by the aunt, who did not give me a cordial welcome. The front room where Séamus slept was darkened in the late September evening. He lay there, unshaven, looking at the outer wall. His breathing was laboured and punctuated with short, dry, coughs.

I went up and said, "Séamus, it's me, June."

He barely turned around and his hollowed cheeks and sunken, dead eyes showed no emotion and little interest. His beautiful hands lay lifeless on the bedspread. There was an aroma of death in the room. He finally spoke as he half-turned to look at me: "Why? I was getting better until you left. Now it's all over. I wish I were gone – there is nothing to live for, not since you left. Good-bye," he muttered and turned away from me.

His aunt was at the door. "I never thought you would

do it to him – not you. He was so sure you would pull him through."

I cycled back to the hospital and felt worse than ever. I knew by then that the nuns found it very hard to get any midwife to work in the Home for unmarried mothers. They would have waited for me. But my boyfriend was genuinely relieved that I was away from the risk of infection. It was with a heavy heart that I returned to my spartan flat. The evenings were closing in and there was a chill in the air.

Later that evening I went to the nursery to look at the sleeping babies and talk to Colette. I enquired about the beautiful baby girl in the large dropside cot. She was nine months old and called Assumpta. Her mother was a nineteen-year-old student nurse who helped Colette with the babies at night-time.

After a few days, I began to take this baby up to my flat and prop her up with cushions on the armchair at my dining-room table. Her eyes grew even bigger with wonder at the strange surroundings. She sat motionless and watched my every move. She reluctantly took a crust with butter on it and eventually put it to her mouth. After a few more evenings, being my only company at my supper, she started to smile when I put out my arms to take her upstairs. It was pathetic to hear her call *"Da-Da"*. It is quite amazing that all babies' first words are not *"Ma-Ma"* but *"Da-Da"*. Ironic in such a place!

I grew to love this little baby and one night, after supper and bathing, Sister arrived and said: "Put this on Assumpta, she is going." She handed me a wool pull-up suit trimmed with white angora on the bonnet.

"Where, Sister?" I asked in dismay. Tears were in my

eyes at the thought of parting with this adorable baby, the only visitor to my lonely flat. This routine was my initiation into the formal handing over of a baby for adoption.

I was told to get Assumpta and take her to the empty labour ward bed and change and dress her. Her own mother was helping in the ward with the newly-delivered mothers. As I took her in my arms, she clapped her little hands (another trick I had taught her in my dining-room). She was all smiles and thought she was going up for another supper.

Trying to put on the new finery was a task in itself as Assumpta kept trying to pull my nurses' badge off my apron. After what seemed an eternity, I had her all dressed up. With the angora-trimmed bonnet, she looked even more adorable.

"Go and get her mother from the ward, Nurse. She must carry Assumpta over the long corridor."

I was appalled at this cruel custom. "Couldn't you just slip her away, Sister – it would be easier on her mother?"

Sister just took the baby from me and said firmly: "Get her mother – are you trying the change the rules here?"

By now I was crying myself. The baby was calling *"Da-Da"* and clapping her hands. Suddenly there was a shriek from the distraught mother when she saw her beautiful daughter ready to go to God knows where. Sister walked first along the corridor that linked the hospital to the convent. The girls stood at the doorways watching this heartrending scene and the mother's uncontrolled crying could be heard all along that long corridor. At the end Sister opened the door that adjoined the convent and turned and took the baby from her mother's reluctant

39

grasp. I had witnessed the horrific ritual that would be repeated for each and every mother and baby in this hell-hole. But this was Ireland in 1951. There were no laws regulating adoption until the end of 1952.

That night I went to my sitting-room and cried for ages at the sight I had just witnessed.

The distraught young mother never slept or ate for the following week. She lost a stone in weight, and finally went back to her London hospital to finish her nurse's training. She told me that she was from Waterford. The matron at her training hospital, who was not a Catholic, had re-addressed her letters home to her mother with the English stamp so that her own family never knew she had had a baby girl during her first year in training.

Life went on. I was learning more and more about the stringent rules and regulations of this Home that was without any resemblance to a home or a haven. I was again warned not to get emotionally involved with any of the patients. My tears the night Assumpta left did nothing to impress Sister who carried out her duty with stoic indifference. Assumpta could have been a bag of apples or even potatoes so long as she was formally handed over. I missed her so much – I could not even contemplate the depth of her mother's grief.

FIVE

KITTY'S SOLDIER

I went to morning Mass as often as I could in those early weeks. I followed the shuffling queue of girls to the hospital chapel and would kneel in the back row and wonder about the three hundred and fifty fathers of the babies. All girls had to attend Mass at eight o'clock – those who were pregnant, nearing delivery and young mothers. Their wan faces and lank hair seemed to accentuate the dark circles under their eyes. They had been up since half-six, and it was at Mass that I first saw all three hundred and fifty together. They wore crocheted multi-coloured skull caps over their short cropped hair.

As far as I can remember, the pregnant girls from the hospital knelt behind the convent girls – the reason I am so hazy about the congregation is the fact that I only sporadically went to morning Mass as time went by for reasons of my own. Some nights I may not have been able to get off duty until near midnight. Sometimes I could have been called during the night for a delivery – so much for no night duty!

The congregation of nuns from the convent had a separate nuns' chapel with a vantage point to the priest and the altar, but where the hospital occupants could not see them. The disparity between the inmates and the nuns that ran the institution became more clear to me daily.

The girls were treated like criminals in this building and there was a general air of penitence. It permeated every corner – even the chapel. Those in charge who ran the godforsaken place like a prison did so as cruelly and as uncaringly as any mediaeval gaoler.

The only expression of love I witnessed there was between each mother and her child. That was mother-love at its best – not shared by husbands. Mother and child were alone and together for at least ten days, at most three love-packed years until the final and inevitable parting forever – amputation without anaesthetic.

Sister and I knelt at the end or back of the chapel. I tried to concentrate on the priest's voice but inside I raged at this regime. Sister's head was bent reverently and I wondered how she could so easily revert to this picture of humility and serenity. I felt guilty for this thought – as if the priest would be able to read my mind. I felt guilty that I seemed to be condoning the treatment of these girls and guilty that I could not accept the rules of the institution. If the priest and the nuns thought that this was what these girls deserved who was I to argue?

And yet, when suddenly one heavily pregnant eighteen-year-old slumped forward and almost hit her head on the wooden seat, I knew that no merciful God would expect this type of relentless punishment. I rushed to her aid, glad that the two girls on either side of her had the wit to hold her until she came to.

As her eyes focused again, she smiled wearily at me and I helped her towards the heavy oak door and from the chapel, noticing the look of disapproval on Sister's face. Walking slowly along the long corridor to the hospital, I chatted to this young distressed girl, trying to calm her.

"The spots came before my eyes, Nurse, I tried to stop them – I'm sorry, we'll both be in trouble now," she said.

"You're fine, pet, don't worry – sure most expecting ladies faint at Mass," I said.

I took her to the kitchen and told her to stay sitting by the Aga in case she felt weak again. After a glass of water, and as there was time before the kitchen nuns were due to return from Mass, I made tea and toast for her. Returning with a tray, I noticed her eyes widen. She ate her toast quickly and I noticed the relief in her face as she swallowed the hot tea.

"Butter," she said as she licked her lips. "It reminds me of home."

I had spread the toast with the butter that Colette usually used. Obviously the inmates were given margarine – the ultimate insult in 1951. Once the others had returned from the Mass and milled around their companion with concerned looks I felt confident that it was safe to leave her and return to my flat. Sister soon briskly ushered the girls to the dining-room for their frugal breakfast of bread and margarine with tea which was served, ready milked, from a huge tea-pot.

I found it hard to eat my own breakfast. When Irene returned for my tray she told me that Sister wanted to see me in the office.

"Good luck, Nurse," she said and I headed down the stairs.

Knocking and entering, I wondered why I was being summoned.

"Nurse," she said. "There is no need for you to leave Mass if any of the girls get weak. Let them go over to the hospital anyway and you stay on."

"That's all right, Sister," I said. "I'd be afraid they would fall on their way over the highly polished corridor. I would feel far happier to come out with them – after all I am employed by you as a midwife."

At times like these, I was amazing myself for being so assertive. I was also beginning to see that Sister could not order me in or out of the chapel.

Busying myself with my duties that day, I noticed that most of the girls seemed to be going out of their way to smile at me. It made it easier to cope with my feelings for my superior! I went to the odd morning Mass after this. Some rare days, no girl got weak.

One afternoon, about mid-October or later, I went to town for my time off. It was almost dark on my return and when I went into my sitting-room for my tea. Irene came in, as usual, with the tray. I saw a card hanging by a ribbon on the wall near my armchair. The message was about all the blessings obtained by going to daily Mass.

"Who put that there?" I asked.

"Sister did," she said. "When you were in town."

I went up and read it again and swivelled it around, face to the wall in its own green ribbon.

"Oh, Nurse," said poor Irene. "Sister will be going mad."

"Well then, Irene, let her," I said. "I do not have to go to morning Mass. She can bully you and the others but I'll go to Sunday Mass from here on. Don't worry – you know nothing. Anyway, what was she doing in my sitting-room? I expect she also inspects my bedroom when I am off duty."

Irene blushed and walked out silently after leaving my tray.

There never was a father who came visiting, or who wrote, for that matter. They were just not around – they had no responsibility. It was surely a case of the girl left carrying the can.

One afternoon a small dark-haired girl came down with her married sister. She was about eight months pregnant. As usual, Sister interviewed her first and when she appeared in the hospital, she was in the usual shapeless blue denim uniform with a smock or apron-effect to hide the offensive bump. She was red-eyed and blotchy from crying and seemed scared. Some of the older girls tried to console her.

Next day, I examined her in the labour ward. I asked her how old she was and discovered that she was just eighteen. I then asked if her boyfriend knew of her condition. She shook her head in embarrassment. I could never understand why most of the girls never told their boyfriends. The whole situation then was one of utter shame and degradation. She was very small in stature and, as far as I could gather on palpating her, her baby was large.

She was very reticent about her condition and told me

that her mother had been dead for years and her older, married sister had reared her and made the arrangements for her to be admitted to the Home as her pregnancy became more apparent. I gathered that the sister had teenage children and then, or course, there were always the nosy "holier than thou" neighbours.

Four days or so after she was admitted, Sister came over one afternoon and called her out of the dayroom. "There is a visitor for you over in the convent. You'd better come over," she said.

There was a buzz of conversation among the other girls.

"Isn't she lucky?" they whispered.

"Girls," said Sister. "get on with the knitting."

I watched them walk towards the convent from my position at the kitchen door. I heard the new girl ask: "Is it me sister?"

"No," replied Sister. "It is the father of your baby."

The poor girl stopped in her tracks, looked at the kitchen door and ran back to me. "Nurse, I don't want to go, I don't want to meet him. Please, Nurse!" she pleaded.

Sister stood and watched the outcry and then said, "Very well, take her back to the dayroom, Nurse." With that she walked back towards the convent.

The poor, trembling girl started to cry and told me that she had not told him and had not told her sister about him and so she was baffled as to how her boyfriend had found out her whereabouts. I discovered later that he had missed her from the area, was not aware that she was pregnant, and eventually found out where her married sister lived. When he enquired where she was he was told about the baby.

He was only nineteen and a private in the army. His mother was also dead and he too lived with an older sister. The poor fellow cycled down to the Home every second day and the Reverend Mother was very impressed by his genuine concern for the young girl who was due to have his baby. He even confided in the Reverend Mother that there were married quarters available for couples with children, and he begged her to talk to his girlfriend. He wanted to meet her just once to explain. A meeting was eventually arranged in the convent parlour.

God help him, he even brought her a box of sweets and begged her to marry him. She was adamant. She would not marry him. But he never gave up hope. As the other girls over in the hospital found out the true story, they were amazed that she would not jump at the opportunity of freedom. She, in her innocence said, "I don't want the child. I'll give it up."

They told her, "Wait until you look into the eye of your own child. Are you crazy? You'll say that now. We all said that until we had our babies in our arms and then those infants became part of us – even more precious that life itself." And the poor little eighteen-year-old who said that she'd give her baby up for adoption was then told that she had to remain for three long hard years and eventually would have to relinquish her child to a foster home.

And all the while the young soldier called with little gifts. The Reverend Mother advised Kitty, as she was now known, to marry him. Then she could go out after the child was born. The other inmates kept telling her to go also, and then one day Sister called me to the office and told me that a wedding was to take place in the hospital chapel.

47

The chaplain was to marry them and the Reverend Mother had a wedding cake made. All was in readiness for a Tuesday in October. Her sister was to be matron of honour, and a pal of his – another private – was to be best man. There was an air of excitement about the place at the prospect of a wedding – the first I am sure.

On the Saturday night, I was in my sitting-room embroidering a table cloth when the hatch was pushed in, followed by a loud knock in the adjoining bedroom. I got up and went to the hatch.

"Thank God you are there, Nurse, Kitty has started the pains – we were afraid you had gone out."

I went into the dormitory to examine poor little Kitty. The bride-to-be was, sure enough, having regular contractions. Helping her out of the narrow iron bed, I put the bedspread around her ample figure and helped her down the stairs to the labour ward.

As we descended the stairs I met Colette, who was on her way to the kitchen.

"What should I do, Colette? Will I ring for Sister?" I asked. I still was not sure if Sister wished to be present for all the births. Memories of the last delivery and the prolonged stay on the chromium commode did not appeal to me.

"Put her into the labour bed and time the contractions – she could be there all night," said Colette.

Kitty was crying now as she knew there was no turning back. We stayed a while and I got the young girl who helped Colette to take the bedspread back up to the vacant dormitory bed. I realised that it was going to be a long haul so I did not ring the convent. At about two in the morning, and after several cups of tea in the kitchen,

Colette advised me to go to bed for a few hours as I would be on duty at eight.

We made tea and toast for the patient and I left her, promising to come at any time if I were needed. Colette, and Celine the young assistant, sat in the labour ward and I left, as there was nothing more I could do. I went to bed and slept very uneasily. It was seven o'clock when I heard the girls next door getting up and my thoughts flew to the poor girl in the labour ward.

Kitty was tossing and moaning with the contractions that were now coming every five minutes. She had a heavy show and was well and truly in labour. Colette said in a low voice: "She'll be hours yet, Nurse. You should not have got up so early."

At half-eight, Sister came over to find Kitty in labour. I prayed that she would not get her out on the commode.

"We will start the bathing, Nurse," she said.

"Nurse, don't leave me please," said Kitty. "I'm afraid."

"Stop making noise, girl, and remember that screaming is not permitted at any time," Sister said.

I followed her out of the labour ward, hating myself for feeling so intimidated by one so cruel. Those babies got a quick bath that morning as Colette was going off duty. Poor Kitty was left all alone. The time dragged on as the babies were fed and lunch was served. It was Sunday, my day off. I could not and would not leave Kitty as I watched the clock in the labour ward move nearer to three in the afternoon. I was praying that the baby would come as I knew Pat was due to arrive to take me out.

Kitty was frantic at this stage as the pushing had started. Sister sat stoically there and offered her no word of encouragement or solace. Suddenly a phone rang in Sister's office and she left to answer it.

"Kitty," I said. "Every time you get a contraction and feel pressure, push and it will make things easier." I wiped her sweating brow and pushed her dark damp hair out of her eyes. She was very distressed. There seemed to be no turning back or no way forward either.

"It's your fiancé," Sister announced to me in her cold tone. "You'd better speak to him."

I went to the office and Pat was all apologies as he explained that he was unavoidably delayed and would not be up until seven o'clock. I told him my situation and it was just heaven to hear his voice on the phone and I clung to the thought that I would be with him at seven that evening.

When I got back to the labour ward Sister had the unfortunate Kitty sitting on the commode with a blanket around her. The pains were obviously horrific by now and poor Kitty was like a trapped animal.

"Sister," I said. "I'm not going off duty until seven o'clock. If you want to go over to the convent, I'll manage here but please don't expect me to fish a baby out of a commode half-filled with urine and amniotic fluid."

She could see that I did not approve of her methods in the labour ward. Kitty could not help shrieking with the next contraction and Sister flushed in anger more than concern. "Don't do that again," she hissed at the distraught girl. "We do not have screaming in here. It is forbidden." She turned and left the room.

I got Kitty off the dreaded commode. I helped her up onto the bed again and she clung to me as she got another murderous contraction. I told her to lie on her side and helped her.

"Thank you, Nurse," she said. "It's easier here. Will it ever be over?"

"Soon," I said. "Very soon you will be a mammy."

It was a full hour later that I delivered a nine-and-a-half-pound baby boy, and consequently Kitty got a third degree tear. Only the lusty cry of the new-born infant filled the labour ward as Sister came in from her recreation in the convent.

"It's a huge baby boy," I said. "I'm sure it was a post-occipital presentation as the head shot out. She needs stitches, Sister. Can I insert a few?"

"No," said Sister. "She is all right."

One hour later after the placenta came and the baby was dressed and weighed, I got two of the other girls to help me carry Kitty to her bed in the new mothers' ward.

"Thank you, Nurse," she said. "I'm not marrying him at all now after that."

Later I asked if her boyfriend was tall.

"He is over six foot, Nurse, and he says he weighs thirteen and a half stone." She was only five feet tall. I don't think that young soldier ever did get to see his son. Kitty was still in the home when I left.

SIX

"SHE COMES FROM WATERFORD"

One afternoon Sister asked me to take some birth certificates to the dispensary in the village. "After that you can go off until six o'clock as the hospital is quiet. If you go in to town, bring back a cake," she added.

I thought that this was the first half-civilised request she had made of me. Her sister was also a member of the order and worked in the convent. They often had tea together, away from the rest of the community, in the hospital office. I knew this was why she wanted the cake.

Following the directions given, I soon found the shabby dispensary building. The mother's maiden name, date of birth, sex and name of infant were recorded in journals here. I never looked at the names or names of the places the girls came from. It was none of my business. I only knew them under their assumed names. Glad to be on my bike once more, I set off for my parents' house on the South Douglas Road, as I had not had much of a chance to go home since I had started my new post.

Once we had chatted, my mother told me that Mr Pollard had met her in town and told her how devastated his nephew, Séamus, was since I had left.

"You could have stayed on – the boy was dying," she said.

I tried to explain how I needed more time off and no night duty and how Pat was worried about my nursing someone so highly infectious. She still argued and said that my father was annoyed too that I had quit my post. This did nothing to alleviate my guilty feelings or my total disenchantment with my new daunting task of being a midwife on my own at an institution where normal conversation or any show of humanity was totally forbidden.

My young sisters were not yet in from school.

"I do not want you to tell the others that you have left Mrs Pollard and certainly you are not to tell them you are working in an unmarried mothers' home. Your father is not very impressed with you either," she said as she handed me some shirts to iron while she went out to talk to a neighbour.

Pressing the heavy metal iron onto the white cotton shirts I tried to control the impulse to cry while at the same time I wanted to throw the whole thing out the window. I remembered how my family had been eager for details after my first interview at the Home. I wished that they had voiced their strong objections at that stage. The meeting with Séamus's uncle, coupled with the associated shame of any connections with unmarried mothers, had obviously affected them.

As I smoothed out the wrinkles in my father's collars and cuffs I thought about the times I awoke with an anxiety at what the day would bring. This feeling almost overwhelmed me. I knew for certain that I had made a mistake and only my Pat's obvious relief at my being away from the risk of contracting tuberculosis made the move worthwhile. At least I also had the chance of going out with him each Sunday.

I had hung the shirts back in the wardrobe and placed the newly laundered sheets and towels in the linen press when my father and my sisters came home. My sisters gathered around me, all excited, and asked why I had not been home for so long. They asked how Séamus was keeping. As usual they made no secret of their pleasure at seeing me and told snippets of their news. I felt bad at trying to play along with the charade that I was still on the private case.

Before I left, we learned that my father was being transferred to Tralee. The girls started to cry – they did not want to leave their school. I felt totally bewildered. I now would have no home to go to on my few hours off. The news of the family's planned departure did little to lift my already dampened spirits.

I said my good-byes and cycled to the village for a sponge cake for Sister. There was a light drizzle falling and I shed a few private tears on my way up the avenue to the hospital gate. I was relieved that I had only two days to go to Sunday and Pat's visit. The thought that all my time off could be spent with him cheered me as I planned visits to films or the Opera House or spins to the sea.

I went straight to the office on my return. Sister

thanked me and opened the cardbox box to admire the sponge cake. There was no mention of reimbursement.

"We had three new admissions this evening. You can examine them tomorrow," she said.

I headed wearily towards my flat and ran a bath. Sleep was slow to come that night with the multitude of mixed thoughts that kept running through my mind at the thought of my father's impending move to Tralee. That night, at least, there was no girl in labour so I got up and went to eight o'clock Mass, hoping that I would get some blessing from the act of sacrifice.

* * *

It was a Saturday morning. After bathing the babies and supervising the breast-feeding, I called the three new admissions into the labour ward to take their histories, record their blood pressure, test their urine and listen to and record their babies' heartbeats.

During these sessions – despite Sister's insistence that I keep conversation at a minimum with the girls – I talked to them and tried as best I could to put them at their ease. Most were more than anxious to talk and to try to find out the rules of the place. The majority of them had been "put away" by their mothers so as not to disgrace the families. This was a general practice in the 1940s and 1950s in Ireland. I must add, at this stage, that all the inmates were Catholic while I worked there and Sister told me once that there was never a case of a teacher being a patient there.

The first two of the three admissions were teenage country girls who had been brought in by their mothers, with their meagre possessions which they were soon relieved of in exchange for the customary garb of all the girls. Both were obviously pregnant and, to me at least, it seemed as if they had to be got out of the way.

The first girl that I spoke to blushed shyly and told me that she was seventeen. She did not have a clue how to assess her dates but told me that in December, the previous year, a boy took her home on the bar of his bike. She was at a dance during the Christmas holidays and she only had sexual intercourse once with him. He demanded it for the cross-bar home.

"I said no first, Nurse but he said 'What's wrong with you? Everyone does this – it's doing a line. I'll meet you next week at the next dance and take you home again'."

I could not believe that this poor child was so innocent, ignorant or trusting with a boy she did not know. I asked if she told him when she discovered her condition.

"Sure, I never saw him again, Nurse. How could I tell him that I didn't know it was so easy to have a baby? When my periods stopped I thought I was run down. It was only when my clothes didn't fit me that my mother got suspicious and went to the local priest for advice. It was he who told her of this place. I didn't want to leave home but my father would kill me if he found out so my mother brought me here yesterday. I told the nun who met us nothing."

After examining her and hearing her pathetic story, I realised that she was almost full-term. It was hard to believe that she was ready to have the child of an unnamed boy after having intercourse with him just once. She went into labour two days later and I delivered her of a fine big baby boy. She too needed stitches, but Sister refused, saying she'd be all right. I think now that at that time, no matter how I tried to deliver their babies' heads, whether it was the commode when Sister was present or pure fright, nearly all the new mothers tore their perineums. Certainly, seven out of ten girls did without the stitches they so badly needed. The glass case was locked and Sister refused the key.

The second girl who arrived the same day was from Waterford. Eileen was her pseudonym. She was a fine tall girl and her baby was not due until the end of October. I remember her labour. It was long and complicated. She went into labour first in the early hours of the morning and, again, I was awakened by a knock on the hatch. By now I was used to slipping on a dressing-gown and helping the patient down to the labour ward where Colette waited.

Colette had something better than degrees. She had been there so long and had so much experience she could nearly tell the hour of delivery by the frequency of their contractions or the amount of their 'show'.

"Go back to bed, Nurse," she said after Eileen had been settled on the labour-ward bed in her calico gown. I palpated her again and listened to the foetal heartbeat and took her blood pressure.

"She'll be there 'til tomorrow," repeated Colette. "Go back to bed – aren't you going out tomorrow? – if I want you I'll call you."

I reassured Eileen that I was just upstairs and told her not to worry. In the morning Sister swished along the corridor to the nursery and then to Eileen, and the usual dreaded commode routine was put into action. Once I had tended to my other duties, I hurried up to Eileen who was pretty exhausted by this stage. I advised that I needed Eileen to be put back on the bed as I could not check the foetal heart or palpate her abdomen in this position.

Eileen was getting pressure at this stage and lying on her back. I opened her legs to put on a fresh pad as she had a heavy bloodstained show. Sister noticed she had a red rash on both her groins (quite a common complication of pregnancy) and said in an audible voice: "Nurse! Be careful! Wash your hands – she comes from Waterford. The quays, you know?" With that she left the room.

I looked blankly at her, not understanding. The poor girl cried out with the next pain and caught my arm.

"Nurse, dear," she sobbed through salty tears. "I was never with a sailor in my life. My boyfriend is a farmer and we are not allowed to get married because I had no money so I had to come here."

"Hush, Eileen," I said. "Good girl, you're doing fine."

Very soon a dark-haired little boy was born. But try as I might I could not console Eileen who found the Sister's remark so degrading and far from the truth.

I was so relieved to have my meeting with Pat to look forward to – the misery of these girls left me feeling so sad, tired and frustrated at my lack of power in such a regime.

* * *

The third admission on that day, as Sister had advised me, with a sneer, was a nurse. I can honestly say that I was in awe of this woman, as she was thirty-six years old to my very inexperienced twenty-two. Her pregnancy was beginning to show, so she had to leave her post as a Ward Sister in a big London hospital. It was with trembling fingers that I helped her up on the labour-ward bed to examine her. She told me of the terrible morning sickness that plagued her and also how the examining doctor in London was worried about her high blood pressure.

Already dressed in the coarse cotton frock, pants and smock, she began to cry when I told her the general rules, and that all babies were reared until they were three and then separated from their mothers if they could not come up with £100 to have them adopted after ten days.

"What form of analgesics do they use here?" was the second or third question that she asked.

I was dumbfounded. Here was a highly qualified ward sister from a London hospital thinking that she could find refuge in this Home of Detention.

"They don't give anything," I had to tell her.

Her immediate and spontaneous reaction was to burst out crying and all I could do was put my arms around her and promise to do everything I could for her when she went into labour. After that, she opened up to me. She was Irish and had met an Irish doctor at the London hospital. They went out together for about a year. As soon as she informed him of her condition, he said that if she was stupid enough to get caught she would have to sort things out herself and besides he was too busy with his career.

In desperation, she contacted her sister in the midlands and both girls came by taxi to the "safe haven". She was devastated at the thought of what was facing her and I did my best to console her.

SEVEN

THE DOCTOR'S DELIVERY

It was only at this stage that I was gradually finding out that, apart from my being forbidden to talk to the girls, or post a letter for them, the girls in the hospital and in the convent were not allowed to talk to each other. They were forbidden to disclose their true identities or even to divulge where they came from. Everything seemed to be cloaked in secrecy, anonymity and shame. The hopelessness and desperation of the place was daily depressing me more.

The girls were getting more friendly to me at every opportunity. Some of those who had been there before I came told me that the former nurse, who had been there for seven years, was on good terms with Sister in charge and never got familiar with any of the girls.

There was one girl in particular – Molly – who waited at every corner to have a chat with me. She was a beautiful knitter and asked me if she could do any knitting for me.

"Get the wool, Nurse, and I could knit a pullover for your boyfriend," she whispered one day. I think by now they all knew the Black Ford Prefect that came up the drive on my days off.

I got the grey wool and Molly started the knitting. She was about six months pregnant, so she used to hide the grey pullover up her smock and take out the pink baby wool whenever Sister's footsteps could be heard. One day, as the latter was coming from the convent poor Molly dropped the half of a pullover back onto the corridor floor. Sister saw the knitting and summoned Molly and me to the office.

I took the blame for this awful breach of the rules. Sister just pulled the needle out of the grey stitches and handed me the bundle of knitting.

"Get on with the matinee coat for the babies," she addressed Molly.

"I asked her to do it and bought the wool," I repeated.

Molly was sent, red-eyed, back into the dayroom and I got a curt "You know the rules here, Nurse!" I must add that the pullover eventually got finished, along with a Munroe spun two-ply cardigan and socks to match – we got smarter!

* * *

On Sunday, as the black car came up the drive, I waited outside the hospital gate in a grey waisted coat and black patent high-heeled court shoes. As Pat opened the door for me he said "Do you know it's months since I've seen you out of your nurse's uniform?"

I had forgotten that all the time I was on the private

case I had no night off. When he would drive the forty miles to meet me I could only sit in the car for awhile with him, wearing my uniform and veil and smelling of antiseptic, while my patient's aunt kept pulling back the lace curtain to make sure I did not go away. Pat had said one night: "It's like the Valley of the Squinting Windows." And now here I was, going off in my Sunday best and knowing none of the girls were in labour. We had the next eight or nine hours to ourselves. This was heaven!

He took me out for a meal and we had a long talk.

"Time on our own at last," he said.

It felt wonderful to be with him again and yet part of me felt guilty for my happiness when I remembered those less fortunate back at the Home.

"You seem sad," he prompted.

And then the words came tumbling out, all the pent-up feelings that only he could understand. I tried to explain how trapped I felt, with my family leaving and not being allowed to talk to any of the girls at the Home. It was hard to describe the general air of doom about the place and how lonely and inadequate I felt, especially in the early hours of the morning at a difficult delivery.

"I wish I could just leave and not go back but then I'd seem like a quitter. I just feel so useless, Pat. The girls are confiding in me and they were warned not to talk to anyone. I don't know whether to tell them that we shouldn't chat in case of further recriminations or risk alienating them altogether."

He caught my hand and reassured me that things should get easier.

"Maybe the rules will be relaxed when the nun realises what a special person she's employed."

He made me smile again – I wanted to hold onto the moment.

On the way back, the thought of returning filled me with dread.

"Are you glad now that I left a dying young man for my own selfish reasons and have, instead, gone to work in a jail?" I asked.

He stopped the car as I was crying, and put his arm around me. "I am very glad that you are out of the infectious house and that you have finally thought of yourself and me for a change. That was no place for you to be. If you just married me all this would be solved."

"I know," I sobbed. "But Mammy said that Daddy couldn't possibly pay for a wedding now that they have the expense of another house move to cope with."

"Who needs a wedding – we could go to England!!"

It was hard to wave good-bye as the car left the driveway and disappeared out of sight. ZK 4865 – I can still see that number plate.

* * *

Two months or so after taking up the post in the Home, my father's transfer came to pass. I cried when the news was confirmed – I, the eldest of six children, always had a great relationship with him. He it was who taught me how to swim and sail a boat, and who gave us twopence in the spring for the first wild flower and sixpence for a scarlet pimpernel in the summer. I realised that I would have no home to go to on my afternoons off.

There was a tearful parting. My whole world was falling apart but I remembered the poor souls that I was looking after and could not compare my situation with theirs. At least now I would have my fiancé to myself and I would not have to lie anymore to the younger ones about my new job. My two brothers were at college and working in a bank and had been fixed up in digs.

"Remember, when we go to Tralee: no letters to say you are lonely or homesick. You made your bed so now you lie on it," were my mother's parting words to me.

I requested a change in my off-duty from Sister. Instead of one day off per week, I asked for two half-days. She sighed as she explained how inconvenient this would be but grudgingly relented. Now I was on duty every morning, seven days a week, and at three o'clock on Wednesdays and Sundays, Pat arrived in his black car to take me out.

As the evenings closed in, my afternoons were very dark so I spent many hours in the large hospital kitchen. This was the only place that gave me a feeling of being at home, with the Aga cooker and the rare aroma of home-made brown bread and scones. I gathered that these were for the convent as I never saw anything but loaf bread and margarine for the inmates' table.

One such afternoon, Sister came into the kitchen.

"Nurse," she asked. "Can you bake? It's a very wet evening – you will hardly be going to town."

"I can, Sister," I answered, "if I had the ingredients."

I hurried to the convent kitchen as instructed and met Sister Phillipa, a nice, tall woman who worked there. I explained why I had come and soon left, laden with a few eggs and margarine, an orange, a lemon and cornflour. I then set about making my two specialities: a lemon meringue tart and an orange sponge cake with butter-icing in the middle and water-icing on top.

Both turned out well and I was invited to join Sister and her sister for afternoon tea in the office. I was told that Reverend Mother had gone to Castlepollard, where the order ran another Home for unmarried mothers. Reverend Mother Therese would be filling the position and I was to be introduced to her in the morning on her rounds.

"Nurse, if Reverend Mother Therese asks you to go to Shannon, say you can't," Sister said.

"But why? I'm not sure I know what you mean," I stammered.

"My sister and I feel like a day out. We are taking a baby to the airport."

This was my introduction to the custom of taking babies to Shannon airport to start their journey for adoption by Americans. I was told that the adoptive parents arrived to vet the babies – one, two or three years old – and then sent the fare along with the expenses for taxis to Shannon.

I was shown photographs which were sent by grateful adoptive parents. But I could not prevent myself from imagining the heartbreak of the natural mothers as their child was picked from the bunch.

* * *

In the nursery on the following morning, I helped Germaine to change Tony. She was a young teenage mother who breast-fed her premature baby son three-hourly. He only weighed three and a half pounds at birth. There were no incubators, so he was literally wrapped in cotton wool. He had lovely straight blonde hair and beautiful deep-blue eyes. He was thriving and gaining weight. One of the happiest memories I have of this place is of that precious baby growing every day.

Germaine was a gentle girl who lived with her elderly father in a fishing village in the south-east. She confided a lot in me when she was so frequently feeding Tony as his cot was near a radiator in the nursery and away from the other babies. Her mother had died a few years before Germaine got pregnant.

"At least she didn't live to see me disgrace the family, Nurse," she said.

I heard talking outside the room and Sister swished in with the new Reverend Mother, who wore blue-tinted glasses and spoke with a very pronounced English accent.

Every morning after that she did rounds, usually with a very delicate little girl – a four-year-old who looked like a two-year-old. She was a mentally retarded child, partially sighted, and had speech difficulties. She was called Mary Teresa and her grandfather was her father. I learnt that the incestuous relationship between the father and his daughter began after his wife died. Now the little girl's mother worked on the convent farm. At that time I had never known that such a thing as incest occurred but as time passed I discovered more and more cases in this place of heartbreak.

Some days later one of the girls went into labour. When Sister was advised that this particular girl had started the pains she advised me that this girl's mother had paid for and insisted that her young daughter got an anaesthetic during the birth. I was to advise when she was nearing delivery so that she could ring the gynaecologist appointed to the Home. I had worked with him before in the university maternity hospital where I trained. He it was who examined me for my final exam.

This was the single birth that he attended during my time working at the Home. Once he had arrived, I administered the ether anaesthetic on a mask and the doctor delivered the baby and afterbirth. He then inserted three stitches in the girl's torn perineum and I couldn't help catching the Sister's eye, as she practically measured the precious cat-gut, as much as to say "this is normal routine practice when stitches are necessary".

After the delivery, Sister and the doctor went off up the corridor for coffee in the office. I got tea and toast for the newly-delivered mother. The odour of ether permeated the entire corridor for the rest of the afternoon. It was an aroma that never returned during my stay there. Later on I got some of the mothers who had older babies to help me carry the new mother to the ward, where she would spend the next ten days with her new son.

I returned to the office for a cup of coffee and the doctor whispered to me as he left "I failed that bitch twice in her final midwifery!" I was not surprised to hear this. I had seen farmers kinder to their animals than Sister ever was to the girls under her care.

* * * *

About two weeks later, one morning at eleven o'clock Sister told me that the doctor had come again, this time to do blood tests on the girls. I thought that, at least, was a humane act, as I was convinced that he was doing haemoglobin tests on the expectant mothers. Most of them looked very washed out and hollow-eyed, with their greasy hair and unflattering uniforms. Sister sent about six girls up to the surgery and, one by one, I took them into the labour ward and sat them on a chair by the window.

The doctor spoke to me rather than to each girl. One of them started to cry when she saw the syringe and rather large needle.

"Oh! Come on now – you suffered more than that for Johnny!" he said.

I was shocked at his scathing remark. As if that was not bad enough, when another nervous girl looked at me beseechingly as he approached with the needle, he said "Too bad about the last one, Nurse."

"I don't understand," I said.

He turned to me with the needle in the girl's vein and, as God is my judge said to the girl, not me: "She died."

I tried to console the poor distraught girl when I put a plaster on the puncture wound in her arm. "Doctor is trying to be funny – don't mind him," I said. I was furious and he knew it. The remaining girls had their blood taken in silence. I made sure that each of them went out the other door to the knitting room. Next day, I asked Sister when the results of the haemoglobin tests were due back.

"Doctor took blood for the Wassermann's test," she answered.

"Are there many positive VD results, Sister?" I asked.

"No," she said, in an offhand manner. "Not since I came here." As if the phenomenon was to her credit. And all the while girls were probably being subjected to the ordeal of these blood tests and being denied the iron or vitamins that their bodies lacked.

After that I thought that any day now the poor girls would be branded with a number or a secret mark.

EIGHT

SADIE'S SISTER

The days were getting shorter. It was November and night enveloped the dying light of the afternoon soon after four. I spent most evenings in my flat sewing and listening to the radio. As the girls took me more and more into their confidence, I discovered that they were adamant that they did not want to give birth under the Gestapo eye of Sister. Between us, we devised a plan of campaign.

If they went into labour on the Wednesdays and Sundays that I was off-duty they waited to tell Colette when she came on duty at nine. She, God bless her, would then put a light on in a disused toilet at the gable end of the building. I would see this light when I returned at half-eleven or midnight and know it was time to go straight to the labour ward. Pat and I would hurry our parting on such nights. This beacon gave some small consolation to the poor girls who were facing their own Calvary.

Very few babies were delivered by Sister after this time. The poor girls often went as far as the waters breaking before going to the labour ward if they thought I would be back in time.

One afternoon, Sister took me on a tour of the laundry and the convent, where the babies of one, two and three years were all in separate nurseries. All the children were in pens or cots and there were three or four other nuns, not nurses, and some of the mothers in charge of the nurseries.

Then Sister asked me to pray for new admissions as the average was dropping. I could not believe my ears. I said nothing. I had far more worthy intentions for my few prayers. She then pointed out that the girls were better looked after here than in the county home. A Hobson's choice, I thought. Her attitude to the Home seemed strange. She had told me again that all the girls here were first offenders, as if that gave the Home a status.

"While there's a man and a woman on this planet this thing will be happening," she said. She also pointed out that the girls' spiritual lives and the future of their babies were well taken care of in this "special place".

She omitted to add that rates were paid to the Home for each mother and baby or that babies as old as ten and twelve months were still being breast-fed by very tired, transparent-looking mothers. This was not the nuns' only source of income. The estate had a huge farm with a herd of Friesian cattle which were milked morning and night by country girls while others ploughed the land with a horse. Glasshouses produced fruit and flowers tended by the girls and sold in a shop, owned by the nuns, in the nearest town. The shop was run by two ex-patients who slept in the convent and cycled to town each day.

In the red-brick building that was the laundry it was dark and humid with boiling cauldrons over hot fires. Red-faced girls stirred these cauldrons, which contained sheets, uniforms and napkins, with wooden poles. There were lines of wet sheets in this building and the windows were high up so no sunlight ever shone in this sweat-house. The girls, with hands as red as their faces, toiled silently with the wet soggy linen and no sound was heard. Sister did not delay long in this place – a few of the girls looked furtively at the "new Nurse".

I was glad to return to the hospital on my own. The following morning, as I passed along the gleaming parquet corridor I saw Sadie, as usual, scrubbing the wooden flooring with a scrubbing-brush which she drew along a bar of Sunlight soap and dipped into a steaming galvanised bucket of hot water. She wiped the excess water from the floor with a threadbare blanket and rubbed until the wood shone like a mirror.

She was about eight months pregnant and mentally retarded. Hearing my footsteps she struggled to her feet and caught and kissed the back of my hand. This was how she always greeted me – her speech was also impaired but she was very affectionate. I often wondered if she were better off than the other poor tortured souls.

One evening shortly afterwards, the girls were in the dayroom where they knitted babyclothes and said the rosary. I happened to be in the kitchen but went quickly to the dayroom when I heard the raised voices. Sadie's sister, obviously six or seven months pregnant and more retarded than she, was brought in. Both girls started crying and had to be separated. We discovered later that the same man had impregnated the two sisters. Here she was, her hair cropped tightly and wearing the uniform.

One of the girls gave Sadie's sister a ball of wool and a pair of knitting-needles. She was like a wild animal in captivity and, as they all trooped into the dining-room for their supper at five, she ran into the kitchen and out the back door. I was in the nursery at this stage and Sister rushed in.

"Quickly, Nurse," she said. "Sadie's sister has escaped. It's dark outside so you will have to find her. I will send two girls with you." In my innocence, wearing only a pair of lime-green sandals, I went out with the two girls into the winter evening. From the back yard we ran into a ploughed field and, when our eyes became accustomed to the dark, we spotted her at the far end of the field.

As the three of us tried to catch her, we were joined by the man who lived in the gate-lodge. At the sight of him, the distraught creature tried to get through a hole in the fence. She was now almost cornered as we all closed in on her. Suddenly, she went for me with the knitting-needles, using them like a flick knife. One of the girls shouted: "Look out, Nurse – don't go near her." It was a most frightening experience as we did not know her name and she was clearly frantic.

After what seemed an age, a uniformed garda walked slowly towards us. The girl was crying piteously and was covered in mud, as we all were. Eventually, the gate-lodge man and the garda succeeded in taking the needles from her and knocked her to the ground. They then carried her, like a calf, by the arms and legs, up the field into the hospital and into a locked room at the top of the house.

As we listened to the sickening sound of the furniture being broken into matchwood and the window being smashed through bars, the garda turned to Sister and said, "Ring the Mental Hospital at once."

Then Sister turned to me and said, "give her an injection of Largactil while the garda is here. He will help to hold her down."

At this stage, I was standing in the kitchen, covered in mud, my sandals and stockings discarded. One of the girls gave me a foot-bath and brought a clean apron and shoes from my room. I was in deep shock, as I had never before witnessed such an event.

Up on the second floor, the banging and roaring continued, which reduced most of the girls and, particularly Sadie, to tears. This, combined with the presence of the garda, Sister and the dishevelled nurse, was too much for them.

Eventually I composed myself sufficiently to venture into the wrecked bedroom and, with the help of Sister and the garda, was able to give the demented creature the calming injection. A half an hour later, the ambulance arrived and the men in white coats took Sadie's sister away. I never heard what happened to her.

*　*　*

Irene, the dark-haired girl who did such a good job of taking care of me each day, was getting very chatty when we were alone. She had the most attractive lisp and would invariably ask me, after supper, if I would have an egg and a slice of bacon for my breakfast. She never used the word rasher.

She talked about her little boy, Seán, who was almost

three years old. He was over in the nursery for three-year olds in the convent and she used to go over each day to give him his meals and put him into his cot at night. To the best of my knowledge, these children were fed on pandy – mashed potatoes in milk – for dinner and goodie – a mixture of milk, tea and bread – for their tea. I was mainly and wholly concerned with the expectant mothers and babies in the hospital.

Irene told me that her little son was soon to be taken away from her. She had heard rumours in the convent.

"Where is he going?" I asked.

She burst out crying and said, "I don't know, Nurse. He may be going to a foster home or to foster parents. Only the lucky ones go to America." I was not aware at this stage that the mothers never knew of their children's whereabouts and that the children would never be able to trace their mothers. Irene was crying uncontrollably now and wiping her eyes with the back of her hand. "I wouldn't have minded as much if he went when he didn't know me, but he can talk now Nurse, and you should see his smile when he sees me."

I thought of the beautiful nine-month-old Assumpta then. I could still hear her mother's screams. And now to think that Irene had to be parted from her little boy of three years – it was a double-edged tragedy. I tried to comfort Irene. I asked if I could ask Sister where he was going.

"Nurse, nobody in here is ever told where their child goes. She wouldn't tell you."

"And where will you go then, Irene?"

"I don't know, Nurse," she said through her tears. "I can't go home. I have no money. I suppose I'll go somewhere – I can't stay here."

This was a desperate situation. I looked at the poor forlorn child of nineteen and was powerless to help her.

"Sister will be over from the convent soon, Nurse – I had better go – Nurse, don't say anything." She dried her eyes and prepared to take my tray.

I was stunned. I felt that I must go to Sister and tell her how I hated the place, I hated the system, I hated the stupid inhuman rules that governed every move I made and, more importantly, the rules that held these unfortunate girls in this godforsaken place.

I hated myself for leaving poor dying Séamus in order to spend some time with the man I was hoping to marry. I now realised that I was privileged above these poor girls who were trapped in this prison to serve out their three hard years of labour and then part with the only person in their lives that truly loved them.

I was going downstairs to give in my notice when I met Sister in the lower corridor.

"Nurse," she said. "You are wanted on the telephone."

I walked to the office and it was Pat to say that he would not be up the following day as he had a bad sore throat.

"That's all I need," I replied.

He wanted to know what was wrong.

"Nothing," I said, aware that Sister was hovering outside in the hall. "I just hope that you will be all right for next Sunday."

"You bet. I'll be there at three o'clock sharp and we'll go for a drive to the sea."

"In November?"

"Wherever you like – you're the boss!" he said.

I returned to my flat and wrote him a long letter that night.

In the morning, Irene brought my breakfast tray, as usual, and she said nothing about our chat of the previous night.

"Are you going to be here for Christmas, Nurse?" she asked with her usual lisp.

"I don't know, Irene – Sister did not say and I did not ask. Anyway, my family have moved to Kerry so I really don't know where I'll be."

"At least you have your fella, Nurse," she said. "You're so lucky."

"I know," I said. "I just wish I could do more to help you."

"Nurse, don't ever say that I spoke to you about Seán – we never could talk to the previous nurse."

I promised to buy a small toy for Seán the next time that I went to the city. This was just a small gesture to help heal the hurt in Irene's heart.

"Seán will love that," she said. "He loves cars – thank you, Nurse."

I met Sister in the corridor on my way to the nursery and she handed me a blue envelope with Pat's familiar handwriting. She remarked, when she saw the postmark, that the youngest patient that they ever had in the home was a thirteen-year-old girl from the town where he lived.

I just said "thank you" as I took the letter. Nothing could shock me anymore about this place – I had seen and heard it all. I went up to my sitting-room to read the letter. In it was a gold pin brooch wrapped in cotton wool – just to cheer me up for his broken date – and a promise that we would have most of the following Sunday to ourselves. I was, once again, ready for the day's routine.

NINE

GERMAINE'S TONY

As the weeks were passing and I was becoming more aware of the do's and don't of this new position I found I was unable to go out for a meal or a film without mentioning something about my work to Pat. Each day off there was some sad incident to relate that he found incomprehensible. He was never inside the hospital door, and rarely saw the inmates in those dark winter days of 1951.

"I knew that it was considered a terrible disgrace for a girl to get into trouble, but I never knew that the punishment went on and on," he said one day. "It's just something that people won't talk about – it's so hush-hush."

"And they can't tell their story – nobody wants to listen. The other day one of them asked me to write a book to tell the world what their lives were like."

"If you live to tell the tale – for God's sake don't try

any more wrestling matches with distressed escapees. I've got you away from TB and then you nearly get yourself stabbed." He could always cheer me up – how I lived for Wednesdays and Sundays!

One Sunday afternoon he told me that his landlady had been enquiring about me as she had not seen me for ages, so we drove to the city for a cup of tea and a chat. She was the landlady who had kept Pat and his friend, another dental student, for the previous five years. It was lovely to go inside the warm sitting-room with a real coal fire. I was always made very welcome here as she and her husband had no family of their own.

I told her of my change of duty. She knew all about "that place", as she called it. When I told her of the misfortunate girl who tried to escape, she was mildly shocked.

"I couldn't believe that the sergeant came up immediately when the nun rang the barracks," I said.

"They never get very far anyway, and of course no one will take them in as a lodger when they see them in uniform with no luggage," she said.

"Would you take one of these girls in?" I asked.

"Are you mad? I wouldn't keep girl lodgers, not to mind pregnant ones. Those girls are put in there as that is the place for them. Anyway girls are always washing their hair and ironing their clothes – I only keep boys."

I was coming to the realisation that there was no escape for these poor girls who found themselves pregnant and abandoned in the 1940s and 1950s.

"Come on," said Pat. "I'm taking you out to Blarney for the evening and we'll go to a film later."

It was like an age since we last met. So much had

as he presumed that she was visiting a daughter of hers in the Home. He told me her name, but it meant nothing to me as the girls had false names and if she was in the convent with an older child I would have had no contact with her.

He was upset, as he hated passing the poor woman on the driveway but decided that "discretion was the better part . . . "

Pat could see that the whole atmosphere of the Home was affecting my usual demeanour. I kept telling him how hard I found it to feel so alone. My position as midwife was very demanding of my inadequate skills, my hands were tied with regard to the labour-ward regime and my overriding sympathy with the poor creatures who found themselves trapped there, forlorn, forgotten and forsaken, was casting a damper on my normal cheerful disposition.

We talked long and deeply about getting married. He was desperately trying to get somewhere for us to live in the country town where he had set up his dental practice. But all to no avail. His biggest fear, at this stage, was that I was being exposed to a side of life that might put me off the whole concept of marriage forever.

As we walked along Patrick Street, after being at the pictures, I yawned loudly.

"You look as if you could do with a good night's sleep, love," he said. "There are dark shadows under your eyes – will I give up my practice altogether and we can go to England and get married and live there?"

I felt terribly upset that night as we parted. Christmas was coming and I wondered if I would have some time off to spend with Pat and my family. His constant letters and visits were keeping me afloat in this sea of sadness. One thing was certain, I thought, as I heard the knock on the hatch as I drifted to sleep – Sister's prayers for new admissions were being answered. There were three to five new patients arriving each week and more and more babies decided to enter the world between the hours of midnight and seven in the morning.

No matter how long I had been up the previous night I was expected on duty at half-eight on the following morning to carry out my duties in the nursery and the surgery. "No night duty," I thought to myself as I pulled on my dressing-gown and prepared to help another terrified girl give birth to a baby that she would have to love and rear until it was three years old and then be parted from forever.

One morning as I checked the expectant mothers I met a tall Dublin girl. She was very thin and pale. I was used to seeing very pregnant girls coming in, seven or eight months pregnant. I had to examine her in the usual pre-natal routine and was curious as to why she was there so soon. As I checked her blood pressure, I asked if her boyfriend knew of her condition.

She started to cry and shook her head. "I started going out with him about six months ago. I don't even know if he was married. I began to suspect that he was when he started asking me if I was feeling queasy in the mornings. Next, he made excuses for not meeting me after work. I was working as a civil servant in a busy tax office in Dublin. Most mornings I had to leave my desk and go to the ladies' to get sick. Soon he kept passing my desk and asked if I had got rid of my breakfast. I just couldn't stand the snide remarks any longer. I was devastated when I found out that I was pregnant so, not to upset my parents, I pretended that I was moving to England for work."

"You look drained," I prompted.

"I am in such a state and the sickness is awful – all day, not alone mornings. I can't keep any food down for any length of time. I lost over a stone in weight already so a priest friend recommended here for the birth. After that I suppose I'll put the baby up for adoption," her voice trailed off.

I said nothing – what was there to say? She continued to have dreadful morning sickness and spent most of the day over in the toilets or else crying.

* * *

Some of the heavily pregnant girls suffered from dreadful heartburn at the last stages of their pregnancy. In the surgery, among the labelled and undisturbed jars, I found a jar of bread soda one day. Two of the girls suffered particularly, and when Sister was gone over to the convent, I gave this innocuous mixture out freely. God help them, it was the only medication any of them got while I was there. At least I was able to replenish the jar when it was going down as a pound of bread soda could be purchased for 3d in 1951. My salary allowed such a luxury!

One morning Sister called me aside and asked me to dress Tony, who was now about seven months old. Apparently, an aunt had called and given Sister the £50 for Germaine's release. Her father had suffered a stroke and was being discharged from hospital as soon as he had someone to take care of him in his cottage. Tony was to be sent to a temporary foster home.

I dressed the precious baby boy who had been given extra-special care and attention since I had arrived and tried to control my sense of heartbreak and outrage as I witnessed the usual ritual of Germaine walking down the long corridor and crying onto her baby's downy hair. She returned, empty-handed, to the nursery, her eyes red and swollen from crying. All the other girls feeding their babies started to cry, and some of them reached to hug her.

"At least you will have the free leg out of this place," said one of them.

For the following week she helped me with the newly-delivered mothers and did odd jobs in the nursery. She was pining for Tony and worried about her elderly father. She got little, if any, consolation from Sister.

The night before she was due to leave for good – Tony was gone six days and six nights – I was on duty alone in the hospital when there was a loud knock on the big oak hall door.

Outside I could hear the rain pouring down. On opening I saw a woman who thrust a bundle, wrapped in a grubby blanket, at me.

"There he is for you," she said. "You can have him back. He never shut up bawling since the night I took him out."

I was shocked. The mite in the blanket did not resemble our beautiful Tony who was nursed with tender loving care.

"Come in," I said. "I will send for Sister."

The woman was inclined to go. I didn't know the

84

procedure but got her into the hall and asked one of the girls to ring the convent. Soon there were heated words in the office. I undid the blanket and took one look at the poor little infant. He was grubby, smelling of sour milk. His hands were even dirty. He had the same clothes on that I put him into for his debut into the big world. When I took off his soiled napkin, his little bottom was scalded and red raw – no wonder he cried so piteously.

"Quick," I said to one of the girls. "Run the bath and don't tell Germaine until I have him bathed and fed – let Sister tell her."

Tony looked as if he had lost a pound in weight and had never stopped crying since he had been parted from his mother. Germaine's breast milk had dried up in the week so I knew we would have to bottle-feed him, probably with expressed breast-milk. Sister went around with a breast pump if any of the girls had any residual milk.

Poor Germaine could not now go home to mind her father. She and Tony were transferred to the convent to make room for the next four or five new admissions. I never heard what happened to her but often wondered if being reunited with her son helped her to cope with the dread of the final parting when he was three years old.

TEN

MERRY CHRISTMAS . . .

Christmas was approaching. There was no change in the daily routine of the hospital. I cannot remember any Christmas decorations or any let up in the relentless, joyless, hopeless atmosphere. The girls carried out the daily chores with the same regular monotony. I was wondering what off-duty I would get.

I had always loved Christmas, but especially the previous three holiday periods that I spent in the hospital where I trained. All the rules were relaxed for the three days of Christmas. The wards were decorated by the young student nurses. We got boxes of decorations and got the patients to make silver bells out of silver paper. Cribs were erected on the big desk inside the ward door. We received fairy lights and holly and ivy from country visitors. There was a prize for the nicest and best-decorated ward. It was my privilege to win it two out of three years. This prize was usually a big tin of biscuits that we shared between five or six probationers, a staff nurse and twenty patients. There was an air of celebration about the place as we sat by the two open fires and played cards with the few patients that were ambulatory and in for the holidays.

We were even allowed to sit by a bedside to talk to a post-operative patient – a gesture unheard of during the year. In the maternity hospital the festive season was even more palpable. Husbands came in with gifts for the new mothers and the nurses. All the doctors gave the staff nurses presents. Matron and the house surgeon carved the turkey and ham in the brightly decorated nurses' dining-hall. After the patients got their Christmas dinner, we sat down and were served by the house surgeons and medical students and we served them on St Stephen's day. We often hoped that there would be no admissions on Christmas Day – of course there always was one, and sometimes two. The air in the maternity hospital was magical with trees and cribs and cards on every hall space and landing and a little sprig of holly on the trays for Christmas Day.

This year, when I awoke on Christmas Eve things were no different than on any other bleak December morning. The only difference was my gold cocktail watch on the dressing table. Pat had given it to me a few days before, with a black velvet box which contained a string of pearls from his sister. His other sister had given me the lovely pink wool cardigan which lay folded on the chair.

I went down to the nursery as usual.

"A happy Christmas, Nurse," whispered a few of the girls.

It was eleven o'clock before Sister told me that I was

entitled to two days off for Christmas and that there was a bus to Tralee, leaving at five that evening, and arriving at half-eight. I was amazed. I could not ring my family as they had no telephone in the new house. I rang a neighbour to tell Pat of my time off.

All that Christmas Eve, I proceeded with my usual duties. Nowhere was there a sign that this day was any different to any other. I had mixed feelings – firstly as to how I was going to get to the bus station with an overnight bag.

I had no presents for my family as my month's salary went on gold cuff-links for Pat. Sister took me over to the glasshouses before I left. I recognised some of the girls whose babies I had delivered the previous months. They all looked furtively at me – afraid to smile and scared to talk. I was given ten amber feathery chrysanthemums to take to Tralee to my mother and told that I was expected to be back on St Stephen's night for duty the next morning. Every time I see chrysanthemums I think of Christmas in the Home.

Eventually I arrived at the bus station and put my bicycle into a store. I got on the bus and checked twice that I was headed for Tralee. There were very few passengers and every village that we passed through had lighted Christmas trees in the windows and some already had a long red candle. I passed through a familiar small village and then a crossroads. I peered out into the darkness, hoping to get a glimpse of Pat, but the hurried phone call from the bus station must not have got to him in time.

Soon we were on our way to Kerry. This was my first visit to my family since they had left. I thought of my sisters and wished that they would be there to meet the

88

bus. But nobody knew that I was coming. I did not have a clue where Prince's Street was. The overnight bag, my handbag and the dozen wrapped flowers made up my luggage as I alighted in the brightly lit streets of Tralee.

There was an air of festivity about the place with shops lit up and decorated and a few men on the streets obviously celebrating the festive season. I walked up Denny Street and enquired how to get to my new address. I soon stood at a three-storey house with six flagged steps leading up to a red hall door. There were cast-iron railings on either side of the steps. A large brightly decorated Christmas tree filled one of the windows and as I knocked on the heavy knocker I could see a coal fire burning brightly in the grate. It was good to be home.

The door opened and my sister screamed in surprise. My two younger sisters came rushing out. The hall had decorations and holly and there was a lovely aroma of baking and the ham was boiling in the kitchen. I was pulled into the dining-room where my father was in his usual leather armchair. He got up and kissed me and asked, "How long do you have?"

It was strange but wonderful to see all the familiar furniture in this rather large dining-room and the usual bookshelves and red polished lino and Indian hearth-rug. My sisters tore off my coat, took the flowers, asked me if I wanted tea.

"Mammy called next door with some mince pies," they said.

I walked into the kitchen and beyond where there was a sun porch. On the table lay the iced cake, the stuffed turkey, and a trifle. How I looked forward to my mother's wonderful cooking!

There were the usual collection of familiar Christmas cards hanging on a string along the long wall of the dining-room. The excitement was wonderful. I was taken upstairs and all three wanted to sleep with me! It was great to be part of a family again.

The sister who was next to me but eight years younger made a sandwich and a cup of coffee for me. I was grateful as I had eaten nothing since my lunch. I apologised that I had no presents for them as I was not sure whether I would make it home for the holidays or not. I gave them a ten shilling note each and this seemed to thrill them better than any present. They whispered that there was one shop open and all three disappeared to buy something.

My father suggested going to Midnight Mass as there was a fine choir in the Dominican church. When my mother returned she was disappointed that she had not been there to greet me. She thanked me for the flowers and seemed relieved when she discovered that I had not bought them myself!

Soon we were in the beautiful Church and the choir was absolutely breathtaking. It was that night that I heard "Oh Holy Night" for the first time. I could not help shedding a few tears and thought of how I missed Pat and also thought of the girls and babies in the Home with no sign that this day or night were so special.

My three sisters were all chatter as we went home to cooked ham and lemonade. My brothers were at the fire, having been out with friends. Soon my sister Paddy and I were tucked up in bed. We chatted sleepily about Christmas and about her new school. As I was ready to drift off to sleep she whispered once more.

"Are you working in a jail?"

"What makes you think that?" I replied, glad that she would not see my blushes in the dark.

"I heard you telling Mammy about a girl who tried to escape and the guards coming."

I tried then, despite my mother's advice, to explain in a vague manner about my new job. She obviously was as innocent as I had been at her age, as most of what I told her seemed to go over her head.

"I saw her that day," she whispered.

"Tell me about it."

"I was walking to Blackrock one afternoon along the Well Road to visit one of my friends from school. A girl – older than me maybe about nineteen or twenty stopped me, asking directions as if trying to get her bearings. She had red hair and a flushed and very frightened face. It was very cold and she didn't even have her coat buttoned. She was out of breath and in a hurry, as if her life depended on my answer. I remember pointing to the Front Douglas Road or Turner's Cross direction."

"Why didn't you tell me that day when I told Mammy?" I asked.

"'Cos I was so scared when I heard that the guards brought her back. I thought I had helped a convict to escape and that the guards would be looking for me. What terrible thing did she do?" she asked.

"Nothing. They were just worried that she would have nowhere to stay in the cold and the guards were the best at finding missing people." I wished that I could believe my own words

Christmas Day passed off very well. The smell of home cooking filled the air and the pine of the Christmas tree in the window added a lovely scent to the dining-room. We played cards around the dining-room table and my Father read. My mother, as was her custom, read out most of the cards – how we hated the sentimental Brian O'Higgins ones! She usually ended up crying into the biscuit tin that held the cards. Things did not change! We went to bed, exhausted but happy to be together.

"Why can't you come here and work in the hospital?" asked my youngest sister.

I thought secretly that I would be a married lady this time next year.

At about five on St Stephen's Day, without any warning, the black Prefect drew up outside the house. I was absolutely thrilled to see Pat – it seemed an eternity since he had come with the Christmas presents. He was all apologies that he did not get my message. The three girls ran out into the hall. "You are not to take her away," they said.

But we left soon for Cork as his flatmate was getting engaged and there was a party in one of the bigger hotels. I made a quick getaway, as the lovely relaxed Christmas spirit of home and my mother's wonderful meals were in too stark contrast to the hospital where I worked. But the adulation of my younger sisters did wonders for my sagging self-esteem.

We enjoyed the party but at eleven o'clock I thought of returning to the Home and retrieving my bicycle from the bus depot. "Don't worry about that," said Pat. "I'll get it tomorrow and bring it down to you before I go home – cheer up, it's Christmas, and think of next year!"

It must have been nearly one o'clock when we drove

up the avenue. Just to remind me that life goes on, the light was on in the upper window. Colette had not forgotten. After a hasty goodnight kiss and "see you tomorrow – I'll ring first", Pat took my holdall to the kitchen door and left.

I was back. Nothing had changed. The corridors were all dim lights. The night nursery emitted the usual odd baby's cry and the usual hush prevailed. Colette had seen the car lights and did not ring the convent. There had been no delivery over the two and a half days that I was away.

"Who is it?" I enquired as I tried to focus on which girl was due. Colette said the girl's name and I hurried to my flat to put on my uniform. God bless little Irene; she had a beautifully laundered frock and starched calico apron and veil laid out on my bed and even the hot-water bottle was wrapped in my night-dress. She made me feel like a queen.

I hurried down to the labour ward and Colette and Celine were trying to comfort the poor creature in labour. All day long, the pains had been coming but the other girls had coaxed her to wait until Nurse came back. It must have been three in the morning before I had the girl and her baby safely delivered and transferred to the ward where there were five newly-delivered mothers. Their babies were in the night nursery so they got eight consecutive hours sleep.

In the morning, I met Molly, who was in charge of the "high dusting" or some such stupid chore. I asked if Sister had been in to the newly-delivered mothers.

"Nurse," she answered. "We hardly saw her. She was mostly over in the convent. Even the babies were not

93

bathed – only topped and tailed." As she saw the expression on my face she added, "I'll get the girl in charge of the ward, Nurse," as she tried to hurry away.

I was rarely cross while working there but I was fuming to think that the poor girls in the ward had not once been swabbed or looked at while I was at home. Sister, who carried out the duties of the hospital with such indifferent precision, had stayed over in the convent with the community of nuns, enjoying the festive season.

I got trolleys of Dettol, bowls and cotton-wool pads and swabs, fresh sheets, pillow cases, night-dresses and we spent nearly three hours making the new mothers comfortable.

"Welcome back, Nurse," they all said as I went to each bed. And to think that a bare week before I had been going to hand in my notice. I was bathing the babies in the day nursery when Sister came over from the convent. She welcomed me back and enquired of my family. I told her of the delivery done in the early hours of that morning.

"Colette did not ring me," she said.

I often wondered if she knew that the girls struggled through the added trauma of concealing their labours until she was gone off duty? I think she sensed my annoyance at the way I found the newly-delivered mothers. The atmosphere was tense in her office where she invited me for a cup of tea and a chat about Tralee.

As we talked, the telephone rang – a merciful interruption, I thought.

"It's for you, Nurse," she said as she handed me the receiver and walked to the door to let me talk in privacy.

It was Pat on the line. He asked how I was and if I had

got any sleep. "Being a man of infinite influence I have managed to get two tickets for the Guild Ball. Ask the nun if you can get off next Saturday night."

I was delighted. I told him that I would have to bide my time.

"I have your bicycle – can you come out for an hour if I go down?" he asked.

"I'll ask Sister – but bring down my bicycle please, as I'll need it."

We whispered our usual endearments and I replaced the receiver on the cradle.

I went out on the corridor to find Sister. She had gone down to check on the newly-delivered mothers.

"There is something I have to ask you," I said nervously.

"Come to the office so," she said and we walked back up the long wooden corridor. Once we were sitting I plucked up the courage to ask her for Saturday night off. She was all excitement.

"A dress dance?" she said. "Have you an evening frock?"

"I have," I answered with a slight pause. "It's a backless in multicoloured taffeta."

"I will put the suntan lotion on your back, Nurse," she said.

I was perplexed so she continued; "I will go up to your room when you have your bath and put on the lotion for you."

This was another side to the woman who could be so oblivious to the plight of the girls in her care. I was stunned – so much so that I then asked her if I could have an hour off as my boyfriend was delivering my bicycle and we could go to the village for a while before he left for home.

"Would you mind taking these to a Mrs Crowe? She lives in a red-tiled bungalow to the right as you go into the village," she said as she handed me a bundle of papers tied with string. "Anyone will tell you where she lives."

I went up to my flat and changed out of my uniform and pulled on my grey coat over the skirt and jumper. I headed for the back entrance to wait for the car. I met some of the girls who asked where my bicycle was.

"It's at the bus station since Christmas – but it will be back any minute now."

One of them, called Dympna, smiled shyly at me and said "We found a half tin of silver paint, Nurse – we'll paint it for you!"

There was not anything that they would not do for me. They really were a marvellous bunch of girls.

Pat and I found Mrs Crowe's house. I walked to the door and knocked. She was all her name implied – dressed all in black. She even had her hat and coat on as she opened the door. I saw a dark dingy hall with a threadbare nondescript carpet running up the middle of it with dusty dark oak stained boards on either side. A naked low-watt (it looked like 15-watt) bulb hung from the ceiling and, as I handed over the forms she addressed me:

"Are you the new nurse?"

I was glad to take my departure. I think that she arranged the fostering of the babies. I never did get beyond the door on my future visits, nor had I any desire to see the interior.

Pat and I went to a local cafe for a cup of coffee. We talked about the dress dance and I told him about the nun's offer of putting tanning lotion on my back. He was going home and expected to be back in his surgery in the morning. It was six o'clock when I returned and Dympna came out of a shed with a blue envelope in her hand and asked me if I would post a letter for her.

I was aware of the rules that I was not to post any mail for any of the inmates or talk to any of the girls either. I explained my position to her and she put the rather crumpled-looking blue envelope back into the canvas bag. She looked so pathetic with her hair greying at the roots and the ends a dyed mahogany brown. As most of the inmates were teenage girls, I always felt especially sorry for those few older women. It must have been harder to cope with the physical toll of the pregnancy in their forties and they were also robbed of the eternal hope of having another baby in a future happier life. She walked back towards the shed and the tears were brimming over her swollen eyelids. I felt like a heel – especially when everything was so rosy in my personal life at that point.

Soon the evening bathing of the babies was in full swing. The girls chatter soon subsided when Sister came into the nursery. She had a breast-pump and went around to all the girls after feeding their babies for any residual breast milk. She put this into a stainless steel bowl and brought it back to the convent nursery for poor little Tony, Germaine's baby.

ELEVEN

SADIE AND FIDELIS

On the following morning, as I passed along the corridor I saw Sadie in her usual position, scrubbing the wooden floor. As I approached, I noticed her stopping occasionally to put her hand on her back. She smiled as I passed but did not get up to kiss my hand as before.

"Are you OK, Sadie?" I asked and she nodded, smiling again.

I went to the dayroom and asked the girls if Sadie was in labour. I was told that she was getting the pains since early morning but that Sister insisted that she perform her daily task of scrubbing the corridor.

My blood boiled. I remember the trauma she suffered when her sister was admitted and the horror of seeing her carried away to a mental hospital. I flew out to the corridor.

"Sadie," I said. "leave that bucket and brush and come with me to the labour ward." As I helped her she kissed my hand and smiled like a grateful puppy. I undressed her, put her into a cotton gown and tucked her into the bed.

"I am getting tea and toast for you now and you will be fine," I said. "You will be a mammy this evening."

God love her. She looked as if she were getting a doll from Santa Claus.

When I returned with the tea and toast the bed was empty. The girl who helped in the labour ward told me that when Sister saw the bucket and brush, she ordered Sadie to get up and finish the scrubbing of the corridor. Several of the girls volunteered to finish it for Sadie but Sister was adamant.

Once again I was dumbfounded. I found it hard to stomach the callousness of this woman, who that very evening was off with her sister to Shannon by taxi to send another baby to American adoptive parents. It was not Irene's son, as Irene had feared, but another little boy called Michael.

It must have been four o'clock when I finally delivered Sadie of a lovely seven-pound baby boy. The joy on her little face when she held her baby is a memory I shall never forget. She kissed my hand over and over and said "Tell Sister that I want to call him Leonard."

As I helped Sadie with the feeding, one of the girls told me that Fidelis had started. I went to the dayroom to get her and as we walked to the labour ward she said "Jesus, Nurse, thank God that old bitch is gone for the day – I am getting the pains all morning but I held on and I was glad to hear that she went off in her black habit. We can relax for a bit for the afternoon. Any chance she'd stay there, Nurse?"

I smiled as I helped her into the gown. As soon as she lay

down she turned on one elbow and said, "Any chance of a dose of bread soda, Nurse? The heartburn is killing me."

I went up to the surgery and mixed the usual dessertspoon of soda in a half-full medicine glass of water. Some of the pals peeped in to the labour ward to see how she was progressing. When she came in she obviously had her hair dyed with peroxide. Now, after twelve weeks' incarceration and probably sixteen weeks' growth of hair, Fidelis looked a sight with jet-black roots and a good four inches of straight blonde shoulder-length wispy hair.

"Oh! God bless you, Nurse," she said. "That's great."

I got the distinct feeling that this was not Fidelis's first time around this particular track. She appeared oblivious to the contractions and was generally very philosophical about the whole thing. I was busy – in an out to see that things did not get too out of hand in the dayroom. There was a hum of girlish talk, which was nice.

Soon Fidelis was getting good strong contractions and already was beginning to feel pressure and involuntarily started to push.

"There's a good girl," I said, encouraging her as I could just see the dark hair of the baby with the last contraction. "You are doing very well, Fidelis – very soon now, in the next few pains, you will have your baby. In fact, I can see the little black head."

"Jesus Nurse, is the child black?" she asked as she tried to heave herself up on her elbows.

I was amazed. "Lie down – you are getting another pain so don't push too hard and I may be able to deliver the baby between contractions."

"Jesus help me," she said as another pain gripped her.

"Could the baby be black, Fidelis?" I asked, knowing

from Sister that she had worked in a guest house near the Cork quays.

Her breathing was more even as the contraction ebbed and she said, "Well, I was with a black man but only once, Nurse."

"It's only the baby's hair I can see – don't distress yourself." All I could think of how relieved I was that Sister was not there. The commode had been firmly shoved into the corner and I wondered what her reaction would be if I delivered a black baby.

Fidelis was more anxious than ever to see the baby so she pushed with all her might with the next pain that she got. Out came a lovely pink baby boy.

"Oh Nurse, you gave me a fright when you said you could see the little black head," she said as she held her son tightly to her chest.

After I delivered the afterbirth and tied off the umbilical cord, I weighed the baby, who had an extraordinary amount of long black hair.

"No wonder I had all the heartburn with all his hair," Fidelis laughed.

He was not her first. While I dressed him she lay back on the pillow.

"Hey, Nurse – any chance of a fag?" she said.

I had to smile. She knew that I did not smoke but kept a packet for another girl up in my sitting-room.

"Go on Nurse, please, while the old wagon is away. I'll pray for you. Thank God it's over."

I returned with the packet of ten Players. I lit the match and she put the cigarette into her mouth and lit up. She could have been the Queen of England at that minute. I opened the window and doors to allow the smoke to dissipate. If Sister had come back early we would have all been in the soup.

* * *

It must have been half-nine that Saturday night when the car lights could be seen from Sister's office. I saw them from my bedroom window and went down the stairs as four very excited nuns came out of the office and into the hall to meet my escort.

I felt great in my evening frock, and most of the girls had gone to the dormitory to get a better view of me going off in the black car. There was a sickening sound of a china vase hitting the bare boards upstairs as one of the girls knocked it off the windowsill. I heard it but I do not think that the nuns did, as they were too busy fussing around Pat, admiring his dress suit, and wishing us a good night. After suitable introductions were done by Sister, we left to go to the dress dance.

It was a truly memorable night. We danced and dined and danced again until half-two. It was as if I had been transported to a different planet. At three o'clock on a crisp January morning we drove up the avenue to the hospital. Through half-asleep eyes, I spotted the light on in the upper window.

"Don't look now," said Pat. "But I think you're needed in the labour ward."

I wearily dragged myself out of his arms, said good-bye, and went towards the back door. Colette met me and said "Hurry, there are two girls in labour and both heads are showing". As I approached the labour ward I could hear the muffled tones of girls in the last stages of labour.

"You won't have time to change, Nurse," said Colette as she handed me the rubber apron and gloves. "It's a long time since we had two ready together."

"How well it had to be tonight," I said as I tied the strings of the apron and went to "scrub up". At the point where I was delivering the first girl, my hair pins fell out and my long hair broke free and fell down my back. I delivered a baby girl and handed her to Celine, who was helping Colette. I cut the umbilical cord and left the artery forceps *in situ*.

Then I turned to the second girl. "One more push and you will be there – good girl," I said. I went to the hand-basin and took off my gloves and scrubbed up again and put on new gloves. I must have looked a sight in a ball gown, my rubber apron and my hair down my back.

I had just delivered the second girl and tied the umbilical cord of a baby boy and was waiting for the afterbirths to come from both girls. Next thing I remembered, the labour ward was swimming before my eyes. The bright lights were on and Colette was speaking to me.

"Nurse sit down, you look awful. Put your head down between your knees."

I blacked out temporarily and poor Celine was standing over me with a glass of water. "I'm fine now," I said. "Just look after the new mothers and carry them to the beds in the ward."

"Will you be all right, Nurse?" asked Celine.

"I'm fine," I said. "Just exhaustion after dancing the night away."

After that I went to my room and changed into my nightdress and dressing-gown. I went to the warm kitchen for a reviving cup of hot sweet tea with Colette.

"I'll tell Sister that you were up until half-six so stay on in bed in the morning. I was sure you would faint before the second baby came. You looked like death."

"I feel fine now. I see that you or Irene had my nightie wrapped around a hot-water bottle – thank you. I'm after such a hectic night, I'll sleep."

The next thing I remember was Sister standing over me at eleven o'clock the next morning. "Had you a good night?" she asked. "Thank you for doing the two deliveries early this morning. The other nurse always called me at night for deliveries, you are different."

"I had a wonderful night and you employed me as a midwife, Sister," I answered. I felt embarrassed at being still in bed at eleven on this cold, dark January morning. Colette had pretended, as she said she would, that I was up until half-six, whereas I was tucked up in bed by quarter to four.

"I'll tell Irene to bring you up coffee and toast, stay on, there's no hurry. It's almost lunchtime. Come down then and tell me all about the dance. You made a handsome pair going off last night. It reminded me of my own young days as a civil servant."

I was more than slightly embarrassed to be still in bed while she spoke. I told her about the dance and what we had for supper.

"There was a photo taken – I'll be looking forward to seeing it," I said.

"Your suntan lotion is still on your arms – it looks nice on this January day," Sister said.

I told her that I would be directly down to the nursery. When she left the room I grabbed a dressing-gown, had a very quick bath, put my hair up under my veil and got into my uniform for the day's work.

TWELVE

BIRTH AND DEATH

I had reached the bottom of the stairs when I noticed Molly hiding near the nursery door. She looked flushed and beckoned me over to whisper,

"I have a bad backache."

"Come on up to the surgery," I said. "I'll examine you."

"I haven't a clue when I'm due, Nurse," she said. "I was never regular."

"Don't worry, Molly, it will be all right," I said.

"Are you on all day today?

"I'd better be," I said. "I slept it out this morning."

"But Colette told us you had only gone to bed at seven after doing two deliveries after the dance. Celine told us your dress was beautiful and you have long hair. My back is aching now but I hope I won't be in the labour ward until after Sister goes to the convent.

I reassured her that I'd be on duty all that day and night. I also thanked her for the lovely grey pullover she finally finished knitting for Pat – even though she was warned against it. By six that night, when I started bathing all the babies, Molly, was in and out of the new mother's ward and was restless. She kept cropping up to report on her progress, but made sure that Sister did not hear that she had started.

At nine o'clock, Colette and Celine came on night duty and it was only after Sister went over to the convent for the night that Molly admitted to having regular five-minute contractions. As she spent most of the afternoon walking around and hiding her condition, she only had to spend two and a half hours in her gown on the labour-ward bed before I delivered a lovely ash-blonde baby girl.

"What will I call her?" she asked.

"Call her Patricia," I said, and she did.

No sooner had Colette and I made Molly comfortable when there was a noise of a car approaching the hospital. It was eleven o'clock – not a usual hour for an admission. There was a thundering knock on the hall door.

"Who could it be?" I said to Colette.

"I'll go with you, Nurse," she said. "God, it's a terrible wet night."

As we both went to open the door, there was another loud knock. I opened the door and put on an outside light. Two gardaí in uniform and a girl who was all wet, covered in a grey army blanket, were on the doorstep. She was crying and shivering and held the blanket around her shoulders but it did not completely cover her pregnant condition.

The elder of the two gardaí took off his hat. "Good night, Nurse, sorry to bother you so late," he said. "This poor girl was found in a well earlier and we were advised by the parish priest to bring her here."

"Come in out of the rain," I said. "I will have to ring for the nun in charge." I took them into Sister's office and plugged in an electric fire as the unfortunate girl was shivering uncontrollably.

"Colette," I said. "Bring her a cup of hot sweet tea."

One of the gardaí took me outside the office door and when Colette was gone to the kitchen told me the girl had tried to drown herself in a well. Her mother was unaware that she was pregnant. They lived in a small isolated cottage, halfway up a mountain.

After what seemed ages, Sister came over and I went down to see if Molly and her new daughter were asleep. I was never present when a patient was admitted, so I waited until I was called back to the office. Sister had a big ledger out and the gardaí were given tea as well as the unfortunate girl. I was told to towel-dry her hair and put her into a calico gown as she had started labour. She was crying so much, she was almost incoherent.

I put two wool blankets around her and stayed with her until she fell into an uneasy sleep. Colette was warned not to leave her alone for a minute.

"You go to bed, Nurse," said Sister. "She will be all right until morning."

I felt upset after what I'd seen. "What next?" I thought as I went up to my bedroom.

It seemed as if I was only in bed for an hour but my gold wristlet watch showed half-seven when I awoke. I thought for a moment that I had dreamt about what had happened last night: the gardaí, the poor half-drowned creature, Molly's delivery, Fidelis's fear she had a black baby, the dress dance. I got up and dressed and went down to Colette who was still in the labour ward with the new admission.

She was getting contractions every quarter of an hour. I checked the foetal heart rate and took the girl's blood

107

pressure. Everything was normal. Soon the other girls were trudging their weary way along the corridor to the chapel. Then they would go into the refectory for breakfast before starting all the cleaning chores they were to carry out each morning. The hospital was shining – all polished parquet floors and high-gloss cream walls with glass and shining chromium everywhere.

The new girl got no name as far as I can remember. Her labour was long and protracted and, at noon, I noticed on her pad that she was pouring meconium (the baby's black motion) and the foetal heart rate had risen to 170 from 120. She was getting very strong contractions but with no advancement. She was very distressed. Sister was in and out and I reported the meconium staining and the rapid foetal heartbeat. Before Sister went to the convent for her lunch I reported that I could not get any foetal heartbeat. The girl was gripped by a continuous contraction and I suggested calling the doctor.

"She will be all right," was the Sister's curt reply.

I was now worried for the first time after all the successful deliveries I had done. This was trouble. Try as I might there was no way that I could get even the faintest heartbeat of the unborn baby. Labour had stopped but the meconium continued to pour like tar. I could not go to my lunch. I told Irene to leave it in the cool Aga oven for me until Sister came back.

The cold dreary January day dragged on until it was dark and then, after what seemed like an eternity to me, not to mention what it must have felt like for the poor girl, the contractions returned. Eventually I delivered a very large nine and a half pound baby boy – white, flaccid, lifeless and silent. No lusty cry, except one of total relief from the mother. As I tied the umbilical cord and lay the body of the dead baby on the towel, through my tears I saw the three-inch band of purple around his thoracic region, like the mark of a garrotte or a boa constrictor.

I looked at Sister. She sheepishly looked away. I got holy water and baptised the dead baby. The afterbirth came soon after and she told the girl that her baby was dead. Word spread around the hospital.

This was my first and only stillbirth while I worked there. I was deeply distressed because I thought that the doctor should have been sent for. We moved the girl to the almost full mother's ward. Soon the news of the dead baby spread and the girls consoled the poor new patient saying "Now, at least, you will have the free leg and won't have to stay in this jail like us for three years."

This seemed to console her as she thought of her half-blind mother living alone. She never saw her baby. The following morning the doctor was called in to take more "bloods" and he signed the death certificate for the baby. His body was buried in a patch of ground that had one cement crucifix, about two feet high, over an unmarked grave. I asked if the chaplain would baptise him.

"No," said Sister. "You did."

The following morning I was doing rounds with Reverend Mother Therese. In her lovely English accent, she was commiserating on the baby's death as being the work of God. The poor girl who was devoid of emotion said "What harm – now I have the free leg."

Mother Therese moved to the next bed. Through her blue-tinted glasses I could not detect her true feelings. Vague dismay, I thought. No doubt the poor suicidal girl could not have relished three years of hard labour and then the final parting with her three-year-old son, not to mention leaving her aged mother.

I never ever saw an hour-glass contraction of the uterus before, but I felt that if the girl had been taken out to St Finbarr's Hospital and had a Caesarean section performed, she would have had a live baby. However, I had no clout in that place and Sister's rules had to be obeyed.

* * *

The pace of the past few days was catching up on me. I longed for Wednesday and my earned half-day. All the past frantic days since the dress dance were just a sign of things to come.

Dympna was haunting me with the blue crumpled envelope and she waited out in the yard where my bicycle was. It was there the pregnant girls cut long logs of timber on a wooden horse with a cross-cut saw. Two held the long limb, two more loaded the wheelbarrow and another two swept up the sawdust and put it in a bag. This was an industry I had not seen before I came to the home.

As if it were a bribe, Dympna produced my black Raleigh bicycle, now painted silver and oiled, with the basket on the handlebars painted red! I hardly recognised my bicycle.

"Nurse," she said. "I'm begging you to post this letter for me. I found out that if I can give the nun a hundred pounds, I'll have the free leg and I'm near my time. Please Nurse, my three sisters out in the world are all nuns and one is a Reverend Mother in Roscrea. They think I'm in England. But my mother is eighty-three and not well. My brother can't manage her. I have a sister who could get my money for me, but she does not know where I am."

"Dympna, you know I can't post for you. The nun told me that the first day I came here."

She looked at the crumpled letter in her hand. "Come

into the shed, Nurse, please, in case she sees us talking. I don't want to get you into trouble. You are very good to us and you are my only hope. I haven't slept for nights and I swear I'll throw myself in the lake one night if I have to stay here any longer. I'll put the child up for adoption. I don't want it. I never thought I could get pregnant at forty-three. Please Nurse, I beg of you."

For the following days and nights Dympna's distraught face continued to haunt me. Her hair had now grown some inches of white nearest her scalp and, with her swollen blood-shot eyes and shapeless figure, she looked seventy instead of forty-three. I tried to envisage her three sisters who were nuns, and how they must have worried about her sudden disappearance. I could not believe what she had told me: that she had £800 in the bank if only she could get word to one of her sisters.

In my innocence and false sense of security in the Sister's involvement with my private life and the obvious excitement she had showed the night of the dress dance, I felt sure that I could talk frankly to her about Dympna's position. Having seen Sister's human side I was optimistic.

I bided my time until one afternoon when I made an apple tart and, as I had a cup of tea with her in the office, I began by saying, "Sister, if you have any influence with regard to whose baby goes to America, I think Dympna is a very deserving case."

"Why, Nurse?" she asked curtly, as I had let her know that I had broken rule number one by talking or getting involved with one of the girls. She waited for me to continue.

"Well," I said. "I believe that she has three sisters out in the world who are nuns and one is a Reverend Mother in Roscrea."

"Yes, continue . . . "

111

"Her mother is eighty-three and not well." I was beginning to think that my voice was coming from somewhere else. I was blushing now as I noticed the stoical expression of her face. I went on boldly. "Sister, how would you feel if you had a sister in the position that Dympna finds herself? Would you not be grateful if someone who could help her did so?"

This last remark did it. The similarity was obviously an incongruous one to Sister. Now it was her turn to blush and it was in anger. "How dare you try to interfere with the politics of this Home," she said. "How old is Dympna, Nurse?"

"She says she is forty-three, Sister," I answered, thinking that she might be softening.

Her answer was measured and curt. "Then she is old enough to have sense. Three years in here should teach her that!"

I was not going to let this argument go at that. I had never contested any of the rules, regulations or omissions of this place with her, but I said as coolly as I could, "I don't think sense has anything to do with how these poor girls end up here. It surely is a question of temptation and 'there but for the grace of God go I'. I firmly believe that any girl who spends any period of time in this place has her purgatory well done."

"Do you really, Nurse?" she asked and there was anger in her eyes.

I got up and took the tray to the kitchen. I had lost that round.

There ended our short-lived beautiful friendship. Things got strained between us after that but I was beginning to learn that the nuns needed me more than I needed them. I had since heard how difficult it was to fill the previous nurse's place. Nobody wanted to work there.

About a week later, I met poor Dympna out in the shed, as usual oiling my bicycle, and I said, "Now Dympna, I am not posting your letter for you. We won't break any of the rules. But, on second thoughts, give me the name and address of your nearest sister and I will contact and meet her."

"Oh! God, Nurse, you are an angel. Thank you. I was at my wit's end. I can't eat or sleep and to think that my life's savings are in the bank and I'm trapped here." She wrote a name and an address on a piece of paper and I went up to my sitting-room to write the "letter of freedom" for poor Dympna. I was now getting used to the inhuman rules that bound the girls to the Home for three hard years.

I got a letter by return of post. Sister handed the letter with the strange handwriting to me with one from Pat and one from my sister in Tralee. I decided to meet Dympna's sister the following Friday in a city cafe and told her that I would sit by the window and would be wearing a green raincoat and a silk headscarf.

As if it were yesterday I can remember, on the stroke of four o'clock a tall, dark, striking-looking girl hesitated at the door and looked around the half-filled cafe. Our eyes met. I stood up and beckoned her over. She came to my table.

"Are you June Goulding?" she asked.

"Yes. Are you Dympna's sister?"

"I have no sister called that," she said. "Is Maisie in trouble?"

She began to cry when I told her of her sister's plight.

"We thought she had gone to England," she said.

I told her all I knew and explained that Dympna was a pseudonym and that everyone in the Home had one. I enquired about the £800 and advised her to come down to visit poor Dympna before the baby was due. We had a cup of coffee and she thanked me profusely. I explained

113

that her sister would have to spend three years in the Home without the £100.

Four days later, in the morning after the babies were bathed, Sister called me to her office. She was very angry. "Did you post a letter for Dympna?" she asked.

"No, Sister, I did not. She asked me several times but I refused."

"Well, how do you account for this?" she said and held out a letter which read: "Dear Maisie, Only for June Goulding we would never have known where you were . . . "

I looked her straight in the eye. "I never posted a letter for Dympna."

She knew then that I was not on her side and I held fast to my guns.

* * *

Eventually, poor Dympna had a baby girl after a prolonged and protracted labour. She called her Cecilia. Like all the others, she had to breast-feed her baby who was put up for adoption or fostering when she was six weeks. Dympna was free to go. She could not believe how much she loved her daughter, despite her best intentions not to grow attached to her.

I met her once some months afterwards in the city and her hair was snow white. If she looked seventy before, she looked like eighty after parting with her daughter of six weeks. Cecilia is out there now – somewhere – a woman of forty-seven years. I never heard from Dympna again and, by now, I don't suppose she is alive any longer.

THIRTEEN

MOLLIE'S ESCAPE

The days of January flew and already there was a great stretch in the evenings. There were several girls admitted and delivered and I was getting more and more used to the routine. At this stage, I was buying ten Players each time I went into the city. There were two girls who used to call to my sitting-room on their way to bed when they saw the light on. They knew that Sister was safely over in the convent and Colette was busy downstairs with the mothers and the babies in the night nursery.

They smoked their cigarette down to the butt and after they had gone I used to open the sitting-room window to dispel the smoke. This was their only chance of a normal conversation since their incarceration in the Home.

One morning, when all the babies were bathed and Sister and I were in the office, an ambulance arrived with a mother and a premature baby boy of four and a half pounds. The mother had stitches on her scalp – about sixteen in all – right across the top of her head which had been shaved.

Sister had a copy of the daily paper, which reported that a woman had been attacked in her hair-dressing salon in Tuckey Street a few nights previously.

She survived and gave birth in the South Infirmary and then was transferred with her tiny son to the Home.

This was Maureen. She was twenty-seven years old and an epileptic. After this assault her fits became more prevalent and prolonged. She was in an awful state of shock and humiliation and cried continuously. I had the most tremendous pity for her as the daily papers were full of the sordid details in 1952.

Maureen's baby son was very underweight and was the only newborn baby that was bottle-fed. Whether this was due to the traumatic circumstances of his birth and the fact that his mother had been beaten unconscious, I will never know. Sister told me to bottle-feed Baby Gerard every three hours. Maureen, who had lost a lot of blood before she had been found, had gone into shock and could not bear to even look at the baby.

All the local newspapers were giving the Tuckey Street case a lot of coverage. It was common knowledge around the city that the mother and child were in the Home. After Maureen had been there for ten days, she was visited by the doctor attached to the Home. I only saw him once going into the mother's ward and Sister was with him. He stood at the door and Sister nodded toward the bed where Maureen was. She was lying down, very pale and fragile-looking. The doctor turned on his heel and I was horrified to hear him say to Sister, "She is a whore."

I do not think I had ever heard that word before. I certainly had never heard a doctor calling any of his patients such a thing. I do not think that Maureen heard him. The doctor and the Sister were in the office for coffee for three or four consecutive mornings after that and he brought down a few copies of *The Irish Times* to Sister.

* * *

Maureen came to me most days to talk about her ordeal. I had to take out the stitches on her scalp.

The epileptic fits started about a week after her arrival. It was at teatime in the refectory and I was in the adjacent surgery when there was a loud crash, and several screams and the sound of girls running. One of the older girls called me. "Quick Nurse, it's Maureen, she fell and hit her head on a table."

I ran to the refectory to see chairs and tables upscuttled, bread and tea spilt all over the place and Maureen lying on the floor. She was purple in the face and still getting the odd spasm. I got a knife off the table, knelt down beside her and tried to insert the handle between her teeth in order to prevent her from biting her tongue.

A few girls had gathered at the door, peeping in and wondering if they could do anything to help. The rest had scattered. I saw Maureen opening her eyes and looking around her in a dazed fashion.

"You are all right, Maureen – you got a wee turn," I said. "Girls, help me to carry her to bed upstairs."

Between four of us, we got her to bed and I put a cold

117

compress on her forehead where there was a large bump. She was very shocked and started to cry. Apparently for years before the assault, she had been free from epileptic fits. She lived with her mother who kept her on a bland diet of mainly steamed fish and potatoes in the hope that it would help her condition. Her father had died about eighteen months earlier.

She broke down and cried uncontrollably. "I was such a fool, Nurse."

I could not help feeling sorry for her. She was a lovely-looking, tall, gentle girl and I think it eased her pain to be able to talk to someone. I felt so helpless. This was only just beginning. As Sister later told me that the case was going to the criminal court in Dublin and that the gardaí and detectives would be coming down to interview Maureen very soon.

The doctor's words rang in my ears. How wrong he was. Maureen was no "whore" – just another innocent girl putting her trust in a man who was a husband and a father and had promised her that nothing would happen to her. He knew all the answers and she believed him.

Maureen's admission and the notoriety of the pending trial seemed to change the mundane pattern of life in the Home. The doctor made more frequent visits. He did not do deliveries, only took "bloods" with the same indifference that he had previously shown. He never failed take a look at Maureen and brought the daily paper to Sister before he left.

At night, Maureen would come into my bedroom. We used to talk for a long time. She found it hard to sleep and the fits were coming more often. She was a total wreck. She offered to shampoo and set my hair. I was thrilled at this prospect but did not want to take advantage of her. Then I thought that it might be a form of therapy, and agreed.

Every Wednesday and Sunday, when I went out with Pat, my hair was shining. I told him about my live-in hairdresser. He had read about the attempted murder case on the paper, and now he knew with the rest of us where Maureen lived.

One afternoon, Pat asked me if I could get one of the mothers and her baby to go to Huddersfield to work for his brother and wife, who were married with two children of their own. After the debacle with Dympna and her subsequent release, I told him I would have to think about it. Sister was often in Shannon with babies going to America, but I had never heard of a mother and baby being released together.

* * *

There had been a lot of fuss and attention from gardaí since Maureen was brought in. Two detectives were coming down two or three nights a week to go over the trial. The poor girl was so exhausted after these sessions that I took her into my sitting-room for a chat when the detectives were finished.

Molly came in one night in a very distressed state. Apparently her father had found out about the baby and was after calling to the convent that afternoon to see her and to offer her or the Sister £100 for her release without Patricia. Molly refused to be parted from her precious baby.

"Take a good look at me, girl, as you will never see me again," said her father. "I'll give you one more chance."

119

Sister was in the parlour – no girl was ever left alone with a relative. Molly said, "I'll never part with my baby." Her father put the ten £10 notes back into his wallet and the wallet into his inside coat pocket, picked up his hat off a chair and walked out of the door, out of her life.

I listened in horror as the tears streamed down her face. I realised then that she had not fully realised that she would have to work for three hard long years and then part with her child anyway.

I remembered Pat's sister's request and said to Molly, "Dry your eyes, I have an idea." I told her of the offer to go to Huddersfield and work as a domestic. She jumped at it.

"Does your mother know where you are?" I asked her.

"No, Nurse," she said. "She is not in good health. Only my father knows. Nurse, I have an aunt who lives in Barrack Street. Maybe she'd help." She gave me the address and I promised to go and visit her on my next afternoon off. Molly left my room that night with high hopes for her escape.

I cycled up to Barrack Street and entered a dimly lit sweet shop. There was nobody behind the counter. I went out to check the faded name over the door. Yes, this was the right address. I went in again and by this time a woman with glasses and dyed black hair peered over the top of her specs and said "Yes?"

I stumbled at first, as I was not too sure if she knew of her niece's plight. I told her who I was and asked her if she would help Molly by coming down to the Home. She listened to the plans.

"I want nothing to do with her or her bastard," she said.

I was shocked. I explained that Molly was going to work for a doctor in England and that her fare was paid. No good. She went towards a door that led into an equally dingy kitchen. She was a disgruntled old woman and I felt that I would get nowhere. Poor Molly. I dreaded meeting her when I returned.

As had happened before with Dympna, on my return to the hospital I went to the shed outside the back door to park my bicycle and there was Molly, waiting in the dark and hoping that I would have good news for her.

"Did you go to my aunt, Nurse?" she asked.

I told her about the uncivil reception that I had got and she burst out crying. "I've got to get out of here. I can't bear the thought of giving up my baby. Sister keeps asking us if the five minutes' pleasure is worth all this."

"Don't cry, Molly, Sister could be in the corridor when you go in. Don't worry, I'll go again next Monday or Tuesday. Be careful, I'll go in first. You'd better not be seen talking to me – we will work something out. Sneak into my sitting-room tonight." I walked quickly away – the feelings of disgust towards someone who could be so cruel and heartless threatened to choke me.

After the bathing session and a check that new mothers were made as comfortable as possible, I went up to my sitting-room and wrote a letter. It was not long until Maureen came in. She had nothing to do with her son Gerard, and it had taken me over half an hour to try to get four ounces of milk into him. Maureen told me that she had to go to Dublin to the High Court the following week. She was scared. She looked shattered. The only consolation she had was that her mother came to visit her every second day and had promised to go to Dublin with her for the court case.

At half-nine, Molly knocked on the door. She had fed Patricia, who was now over twelve weeks old and getting more beautiful each week.

"Nurse," she said. "When I came in here I had saved up £32 in a post office account. When my aunt gets me out of here tell her I'll give it to her if she lets me go into the post office to sign. She could say that she will give me and the baby a home." God help her, she seemed all keyed up at the thought of going to England and making a new life for herself and her baby.

I promised that I would try and visit the aunt again and pass the message on about the £32.

"My aunt has drink problem, Nurse – that £32 would mean a lot to her," she then whispered.

As if I had not guessed that the first day I called.

* * *

I am sure that there were three more dress dances around this time. Each time, Sister was very excited and offered to put the tan lotion on my back, and each time she brought four nursery nuns over to see Pat and me going off. It was extraordinary to me that she could be one person with me and then the very opposite to those in her care. Then again, when I thought of Molly's father and her aunt, I wondered if I were the strange one to doubt that the punishment should be so severe for such a human crime.

One morning, I went down and was told by one of the mothers that Molly and her baby had been sent over to the convent. I was shocked. I had no way of managing a meeting with Molly now.

But as promised, I went to Barrack Street again and this time I found the aunt in a more agreeable mood. The promise of the £32 did the trick, plus the fact that she was not expected to have anything to do with her misfortunate niece in the future.

One afternoon, as I was going to the kitchen, a dark-haired girl who had a two-year-old daughter in the convent stopped me with a furtive look over her shoulder. She beckoned to me to take a note from her hand, keeping an eye on the corridor for Sister's footsteps. It was from Molly, written in pencil. I was to give a note to this girl and she was to put it in a hole in the convent wall. Molly sounded desperate.

I was half afraid of writing anything after the letter to Dympna's sister, but there was no other way we could now communicate. I wrote a note and mentioned no name and signed nothing. Molly would know. The aunt was coming on the following Friday week. I warned the dark-haired girl to be careful.

"Don't worry, Nurse," she said. "I will."

* * *

I think this period in the Home was the most hectic. I had made contact with Molly's aunt but now that the cranky old woman had consented to go to see her niece, it was frustrating and worrying to have poor Molly banished to the convent. This was a complication I had not reckoned on and I was scared for Molly's sake that we would be found out. I still can remember the anger in Sister's face when she opened and read the letter about Dympna that mentioned my name.

Maureen's High Court case was getting closer. Two detectives were at the Home taking statements two or three nights a week. She came up to the dormitory looking worn out after these sessions. One thing was certain, she could not have inflicted the head wound herself.

Every other afternoon, just as lunch was over, the girl in the kitchen had a note from Molly and I sent over one on the latest developments with her aunt. It was a most difficult time as I knew the rules, and the contact with England was only by letter. Things were very up in the air and then there was the question of Sister, who was not often away.

One afternoon, Sister told me she and her sister were going to Shannon again with a baby who was going to America. These children were the chosen few and the lucky ones, according to Sister. I was able to go to Molly's aunt to tell her to be ready to collect Molly and her baby on a particular Friday. Then I had to hide a note to tell Molly about this arrangement. I also had to write to Huddersfield to confirm that Pat's brother should go to Liverpool to collect Molly and little Patricia.

I heard from one of the girls that one of the elderly nuns had signed the register for Molly and the aunt. Molly was seen grabbing a blanket to wrap around her sleeping baby and running quickly from the building to the waiting car. She had told this girl that her aunt had organised for one of her cousins to drive her to the boat in Dublin.

Sister never mentioned anything about Molly and

Patricia's departure. I waited frantically for news. Molly must have been afraid to write to me at the Home. Two weeks later, Pat told me that one of his sisters had received a letter from Huddersfield, confirming that the Irish girl and her baby were well settled in. It was not until many years later – 1990 in fact – that I heard the story.

Maureen's case was in *The Irish Times*. The doctor came down two days in succession with a copy of the paper for Sister. I was excluded from this "club". They had coffee in her office and I looked after the mothers and babies.

It must have been around this time that Irene came over one morning with my breakfast, with her face swollen and red. As soon as I saw her I knew that Seán had gone. She was beside herself. What could I say? She did not know where her baby boy of three was gone, and he had been just as upset at being wrenched from his mother the night before.

I knew I had no business asking Sister for any information and I also knew that I was on thin ice since Molly's departure. I just concentrated on the daily routine. When Maureen came back from Dublin she brought me a beautiful gold brooch with ivy leaves etched in an oblong frame. Her attacker, the father of her baby son, got seven years in jail.

I do remember that she asked me to get wool as her mother wanted to knit me a twin set for all I had done for her daughter. She stayed on there for four months. The baby, who had a congenital heart problem, was transferred to St. Finbarr's Hospital as soon as we got his weight to eight pounds. Maureen's mother posted me the beautiful hand-knit twin set. Eventually the epileptic fits became so frequent that Maureen was sent to Moorepark, a home for epilepsy sufferers.

* * *

My Sundays and Wednesdays were very precious to me. Every week we had some very sad cases and there was always one more tragic than most. One afternoon, Sister asked me to take a four-month-old baby to Dublin on the train. The mother was a sixteen-year-old girl who had gone to mind her sister's three children while she went into hospital to have her fourth baby. Her brother-in-law got her pregnant, and the poor child was warned by her mother not to tell her sister. The mother brought her from County Meath to the Home.

A taxi was to collect me and the baby at seven to bring us to the eight o'clock train for Dublin. The baby was dressed in pink and wrapped in a pink shawl. Sister gave me £10 to cover my expenses for the day.

I got as far as Mallow before the baby girl woke. I had been given a bottle of milk before I left. For most of the journey to Dublin the poor infant cried and cried. The guard heated the bottle twice for me, but no way would the baby take the bottle. The other occupants in the carriage enquired if it was my first. I walked out on the corridor and up and down and still the poor mite kept crying.

I was dressed in my ordinary clothes so nobody knew but that I was the baby's incompetent mother! The guard was very kind and heated the bottle once more, but the baby would not take it. I went to the toilet and rocked her over and back and this pacified her for a while but, for most of the journey, she was fretful and I was totally embarrassed.

At the Dublin station, I saw the familiar face of a girl that I had trained with. She was a native of Dublin and took the baby from me.

"I wish I had a camera," she said. "With her colouring nobody would believe that she was not Pat's!"

I told her that I was to get a taxi to take the baby to the Irish Sisters of Charity in Blackrock.

"Don't mind the taxi," she said. "We'll get the bus. It's not far."

Soon we were at the big hall door of the orphanage and the baby started to cry again. I rang the bell. It was eventually opened by a nun. I told her where I had come from. She led us into a parlour along a highly polished corridor with statues and holy pictures lining the two sides. The parlour had a long table with six mahogany straight-backed chairs and more statues with red and blue night-light covers at the foot of the Sacred Heart and Our Lady.

The nun tiptoed out of the room and the baby started to cry louder when I sat down. We must have been there ten minutes and the baby was in a frenzy when eventually this figure in a black habit with a silver crucifix on her chest came in.

"What is wrong with the baby?"

Above the cries, I said, "I think she is hungry, Sister, but she won't take the bottle." I tried to explain that the baby was fully breast-fed and had been last fed at six that morning.

"*What?*" shrieked the nun. "Why wasn't she weaned? They knew she was to come here!"

Above the wailing of the baby it was very hard to make oneself heard. My friend, who saw that I was embarrassed and exhausted, interrupted. "Why don't you ring the Home and talk to the nun who sent her here?"

That seemed to stun the tall nun into silence. "Give her to me," she said as she grabbed the poor baby and took the bottle. She disappeared out into the corridor.

"Come on – you look like someone who could do with a nice lunch," said my friend as we left. We chatted and ate our lunch and got a bus back to the train. I slept nearly all the way home. It made a change from the stressful journey up. I was glad to get a taxi from the train to the Home and went straight to bed.

That little baby girl's cries were still being replayed in my mind and I could not help wondering how the hungry little thing was managing. That was the only occasion that I was asked to take a baby anywhere.

FOURTEEN

MARIE THE REBEL

The afternoon that Marie arrived, there was terrible commotion up in the Sister's office. The new admissions were always received in the convent parlour and they were led to believe that they had arrived at a "rest home". The initiation to the Home and the stripping of all outside clothes took place after the girls' mothers had gone.

Marie was different. She was from Dublin, eighteen years old. Her father was a colonel or a commandant in the army. Her mother was about forty – a silly woman according to Sister – and she had driven Marie to the Home and handed over the £100 so that Marie could go back home or to boarding school when her baby was ten days old.

Marie screamed that she would not put on that awful uniform and would not part with her colourless nail varnish or her jar of Ponds vanishing cream. Sister had to intervene. She told Marie she was no different to any of the girls who were already there and also added "It is the same thing that has landed you all in here."

Marie wailed for her mother and it must have taken an hour or more to calm her down. Her face smudged with tears, she ran up to me – as if I could help her. She would not take the ball of wool and the two needles offered to her in the dayroom.

"Nurse," she said. "I can't knit and I am not going to try. I'm out of here in twelve weeks."

God love her, I thought. Her pregnancy was showing and she was in for a rude awakening. She gave the height of cheek to Sister and would not conform. Half the time she was looking out the window or running up to me in the day nursery.

At that particular time, a priest, a Father Hegarty, was trying to get a baby with a good background for a family to adopt out in the city. Marie was sent for very often to be questioned about the father of the baby. She closed up like a clam and would not tell either Sister or Father Hegarty about her boyfriend or anything else.

It seemed she had a boyfriend. He used to write to her and send her presents – a string of pearls and material for frocks, as he worked in a city fashion store. She used to come into my sitting-room at night and on one occasion told me how she got pregnant. She and another girlfriend went to a party. There she met an Englishman who brought her a drink or gave her a drink, and the next thing that she knew, she woke up in his apartment the following morning, in his bed.

He drove her home. She pretended she had spent the night with her school-friend. She thought that this was all great experience and thought no more of it until two months went by and she got no period. She felt very sick in the mornings. One evening she met the Englishman again, going into a hotel. She went up to him.

130

"I'm pregnant."

"You are old enough to take care of yourself," he said.

She was horrified. She was sure he'd offer some suggestion. He just walked off and left her standing in the street.

A few nights later, when out with her boyfriend, she broke down and told him what happened at the birthday party. He was horrified, but being the sensible lad that he was, he said, "You will have to tell your mother. I'll go with you. She'll help – you can't go on like this. Don't worry, I'll stand by you."

It seemed to give her some comfort to unburden herself to me. I found it difficult to believe that a young girl of eighteen would even contemplate going out with an older man, not to mind accepting a drink or going to his flat. It was beyond my limited imagination in 1952.

Marie was now plagued by Sister and Father Hegarty as to the identity of the father of her child. She would not and did not tell her story to anyone but me. Needless to add, I kept her secret. I was not even supposed to talk to the girls, let alone entertain them in my sitting-room.

Sister confided in me one evening that Father Hegarty was trying to get a baby from a nice background for these friends who wanted to adopt a baby. Marie's boyfriend sent three yards of material most weeks to her and then a purple velvet box of pearls. Sister was sure that this nice Irish boy was the father of the expected baby.

I think the fact that Marie's father was an officer in the army influenced Sister with regard to the baby's pedigree. I kept my thoughts to myself. It had nothing to do with me. I tried once for Dympna's sake to interfere and where did it get me?

131

Marie grew daily more truculent. She refused to mix or talk with any of the girls. No way would she learn to knit. She followed me around the hospital and every night I was in my flat, she came in for a chat.

* * *

One afternoon, a schoolgirl of fifteen with long hair down to her waist wearing the Brigideen navy uniform was admitted. Her mother brought her in and gave £100 to Sister as she, the schoolgirl, was the youngest of eight children and her father was a farmer from County Meath.

The mother was distracted. She had taken the girl to their local GP at the Easter holidays as she had acne, mostly on her forehead. After ten minutes with the child, he came out to the waiting room and asked the mother to come to the hall.

"Do you realise that your child is seven months pregnant?" he asked. Apparently the young farmhand had been coming in through a window of the ground-floor bedroom the girl shared with an older sister. He came when the older sister was out, gave her sweets and told her to tell nobody.

The mother was devastated. If she told her husband the truth, he would have taken down the shotgun from over the fireplace and blown the farmhand's head off as the youngest girl was his pet. There was no excuse to fire him as he was a willing worker and the worst part for the woman was that she had to serve him three meals a day.

This new admission, who became known as Julie, intrigued poor Marie and the two of them became friendly. Both girls were lucky that their mothers had paid

132

for their freedom, but they would still have to part with their babies.

Marie was the first to go into labour. After a relatively trouble-free twelve hours, she was safely delivered by me of a baby boy. She called him Albert Victor and breast-fed him for the ten days.

I was asleep when Marie came into my bedroom one early morning, dressed in a beautiful green tweed coat over a beige polo neck jumper and green pinafore. She woke me to say good-bye and thanked me and asked me what would she do with her breast milk?

"Ask your Mum – don't drink too much," I said.

She cried as she hugged me and whispered, "I'll miss him. I love him."

She was gone in a flash. Before I left to get married in June, I read an announcement in *The Cork Examiner*. "Darling child of Mr & Mrs . . . , Albert Victor, died suddenly." Marie never knew that her little son did not live to see a mid-summer's day.

When Marie left, there was a void. Every day had brought fresh drama with her. Although she was only eighteen, I admired her guts. She tried her mighty best to buck the system.

* * *

One night Colette developed a terrible toothache. A dentist did come out and did extractions for about ten or twelve of the girls, but it emerged that Colette needed multiple extractions. A doctor came one morning, and gave her an anaesthetic as the dentist removed all her upper and lower teeth.

I got some of the more senior mothers to help me to take her up to the bedroom on the corridor leading to my flat. I never knew where Colette slept. The room had a three-foot iron bed, a white bedspread, a small wardrobe and a locker with a bare wooden floor. No curtains – oil-painted gloss in cream was all that decorated the walls.

We got her into her nightdress and I brought a towel from my bedroom and got a second pillow and covered it with a towel. I left a receiver for her to spit into. I kept an eye on her all the afternoon and at four, I cycled to the village for two packets of Marietta biscuits and came straight back. She dozed most of the afternoon and Sister said that she could take the night off – after twenty-four extractions?!

Celine and another girl were on night duty and I was in for the following two nights so all was quiet, only for the whimpering new babies beneath in the night nursery. I brought up tea and allowed it to cool for Colette to drink. I gave her the biscuits to dunk in the cool tea and I slipped her two Anadins from my own supply. She was very grateful, and I promised to be in later and get more tea. The hospital was quiet. No cases were imminent so I could devote some time to poor Colette.

I knew enough about dental nursing (after all that was where I met Pat – in the dental hospital – not an overly romantic place!) not to give her any mouthwashes for twenty-four hours. I also suggested to Sister that she would need at least one other night off as she had lost a good deal of blood. I told Sister that I would be on call and would not leave the hospital until the following Sunday.

Sister allowed Colette the luxury of two consecutive nights in bed for her thirty years of service. The Marietta biscuits were all the solid food she had for days. I got soup and Bovril from Sister Phillipa in the kitchen. Colette said that she would be eternally grateful to me. After that there were many more nights in the Hospital kitchen where Pat and I had tea and hot buttered toast after a date.

* * *

Spring was in the air. The birds were singing. The shrubs were a mass of blossoms and the long dark evenings were stretching into longer days. Pat told me one night of a dental dinner that was being held by one of his professors who was president of the Dental Association.

I told Sister about the dinner and, as usual, she showed great interest and asked what I was going to wear.

"I suppose I'll wear my evening or dress-dance frock."

"The backless one?" she asked.

"Yes," I said. "I have only that one or my white."

"You can't go to a dinner unless you wear a dinner-gown with long sleeves," she said. "I'll get Sister Cyril to make you one. She is a marvellous dressmaker. This is great. It brings back memories."

One night soon afterwards, she called me to the office after the bathing. She was in high good humour. "Nurse," she said. "I have told Sister Cyril about the coming dental dinner and she has agreed to make a gown for you. Tonight at nine o'clock, I have asked her to call over to measure you and talk about the material and how many yards you need to buy."

Naturally, I was delighted and taken aback. My mind started to race about the price of the material and I wondered if my salary would stretch that far. Shortly after nine, Sister Cyril arrived – a tall well-proportioned nun with a jolly laugh, and very direct. "Get a Vogue pattern," she said. "No other one will do. If you don't get a Vogue pattern I won't guarantee a successful gown. All I want in return is a box of Morny French Fern soap," she added.

"Tell Nurse how many yards to buy," said Sister.

"I'll measure you – usually for a full-length gown you'd need five yards of 36" wide," said Sister Cyril. "Don't forget now, a Vogue pattern. I'll see you on Friday night after Reverend Mother puts out her light – I'll sleep over here."

I thanked her and left the two in the office. I had never seen Sister in this new mood before. Neither had I been to four dress dances and now a dental dinner in one year!

* * *

There was a gentle rain the next day so I stayed in my sitting-room doing embroidery. One of the girls crept up to find me to tell me that there was a terrible commotion in the dayroom.

"Where is Sister?" I asked, as officially I was off duty and not supposed to have anything to do with the girls while they were knitting.

"I think the last girl who was admitted this morning is from the same town as four other pregnant girls, Nurse."

I put away my embroidery and walked along the top corridor with her.

As we neared the top of the stairs that was directly over the dayroom I asked why there was such a fuss.

"As far as I know, the four girls from Macroom knew that there was another girl in trouble. They knew that

136

they had been with a particular young fella of twenty and now they know that this girl was with him, too."

As I entered the room there was sheer bedlam. All five girls were crying and calling each other names. The girl who had called me was afraid that there was going to be a riot as things were flung and hair was pulled. The biggest fear was that Sister would come over from the convent and witness the commotion. As soon as one of them noticed me and beckoned to the others, there was silence. The newly-admitted girl, who was red-faced and crying, went off on her own to a corner.

I was also in a state of shock as I knew perfectly well that Sister would not tolerate this outburst of emotions for one minute. None of the girls were supposed to talk to each other or to me. Little by little the babble subsided.

"You know, girls," I said, "Sister won't stand for any of this carry-on."

One of the girls said it was all the new girl's fault. "So smart Frank fooled you too?" This comment was directed at the new admission.

It surely must have been very humiliating for her to see four very heavily pregnant girls from her own home town, and then to be told that the one young man had been responsible for all five pregnancies.

"I suppose he told you he'd marry you too, like he told us poor fools? We all thought that you'd be smarter – with your airs and graces around the dance hall."

I interjected at this point as I could see a big row developing again. Most of the older girls and the new mothers tried to restore order. One said, "You'd better be quiet as Nurse will get into big trouble if Sister comes over."

I asked the new girl to come to the surgery to take her

particulars and check her blood pressure. I knew that Sister would not be over for another hour or so. This upset was a new and uncomfortable position for me. After about ten minutes the poor girl settled down and I told her a few of the rules. At this stage parting with her unwanted baby was the least of her troubles. I knew from experience that would change totally once she looked into her own child's eyes. She seemed very upset at the thought of remaining imprisoned at the Home for three years.

Very soon there was peace again. I heard the girls going into the dining-room for their tea. I went in and asked three of the more senior girls if this new girl could sit at their table. They were quite agreeable and the rest of the day passed off uneventfully. I thought of the twenty-year-old boy who had got five girls into trouble in the space of a few months. No doubt but it was a man's world.

By the time Sister came over for the bathing and feeding that night, all appeared calm in the dayroom. Once the routine had been completed Sister asked me to call to the office for a minute.

She told me how shocked she was when the mother of the new admission explained that it was rumoured the there were four others already at the Home who had been made pregnant by the same young man. Of course Sister blamed the girls for being so free with their favours.

I did not let on what had happened earlier and felt surprised that she told me anything about the situation at all. I was glad to have been able to diffuse some of the tension that had been in the room that day and I wondered if that young man would ever know how much pain and sorrow he had caused with his predatory charm and empty promises.

FIFTEEN

SISTER CYRIL'S DINNER-GOWN

The Hospital was quiet on the following day. As I looked out the window, another admission could be seen trudging up the long avenue. She was obviously pregnant by her walk, carried two brown cases and was all alone. I waited until Sister had taken all her particulars and possessions and handed her over to a senior mother to help her into the uniform.

She sheepishly walked up to the dayroom and I met her on the corridor. I was just going up to my flat to change out of my uniform but I stopped to welcome her and explained that I would see her first thing in the surgery on the following morning. She looked older than the others. I took a rough guess that she was about seven months pregnant.

Within fifteen minutes, I was on my way into the city for a pattern, material and a matching reel of thread. I headed for Dowden's, the most exclusive shop in the city, and prayed that I would have enough money. Pouring over diagrams of evening frocks in the big pattern book, I chose an ice-blue crepe material and the most beautiful Vogue pattern with a double cape effect and not too low a cleavage, seeing as a nun was making it!

I brought a cake for supper that night. Sister was partial to Green Door confectionery and I dearly wanted to stay in her good books. I had broken a good few of the rules and at least I had secured the release of one girl with her baby to my future brother-in-law in Huddersfield. I had also helped poor Dympna by going to meet her sister.

I cycled back with my purchases. It was lovely to have the lengthening evenings again and to hear the birds singing. I called to the small shop for the usual Players for the few girls that smoked. After I had the babies sorted that evening, I checked the newly-delivered mothers and then returned to my flat. I wrote a quick letter to Pat, telling him about the dinner-gown. It was barely ten days away but Sister Cyril assured me that she would have it ready in a week with only one fitting!

I felt so excited at the thought of the new frock and yet felt guilty when I remembered how badly torn those new mothers were. They rarely complained, but their discomfiture was so obvious as they tried to feed their babies without sitting up. I remembered those women who complained that their stitches were pinching them in the training hospital – I could not imagine the pain of being torn and never repaired.

There were times when I could work routinely from day to day and cling to the moments when Pat came. There were times when the camaraderie of the girls kept our spirits up even though it was forbidden. Most of the time I was trying to struggle with my urge to stop all this daily misery. Surely these girls had suffered enough by being rejected by the fathers of their babies, their families, the neighbours and society in general without the added torture of being made to go through the savage customs of this place?

There was a knock on the door of my sitting-room. It was the girl Pauline who "would kill" for a fag!

"Nurse," she said. "Any chance of a puff? I saw you going away this evening."

I gave her the cigarette and the matches and said, "Go over to the toilet at the gable and lock the door. Open the window and mind the butt in case Sister comes up to my flat. Here – take two cigs and be sure to flush the butts down the loo."

"Thanks, Nurse," she said. "I'll say a prayer for you."

I took my material, pattern and cake down to the office and, as it was vacant, I left them on the desk. Sister Cyril did say that she had to wait until Reverend Mother was asleep – she could see the shaft of light under the split in the door. So the nuns were capable of breaking a few rules too! This thought gave me a little comfort. I wondered if the new admission had gone to bed or was still in the dayroom knitting?

I went up to the night nursery to Celine and Colette, who was looking a small bit better after her recent dental extractions.

It must have been after ten o'clock when the two nuns came over from the convent and I was sent for. Sister Cyril was in her nightdress with her black habit over it. Her bare feet were in wine velvet slippers. Sister was still in her white nurse's habit. They were more excited to see the cake than my choice of ice-blue crepe. Sister Cyril took out her measuring tape and her red memo notebook.

"I'll do the measuring of Nurse's statistics," she said. "You go and make a pot of tea."

It was a welcome change to meet someone so natural and so spontaneous and always ready with the jolly remark. She had an infectious laugh. She joked about my boyfriend and how good he was to take me to all the dress dances and now a dinner.

Once we had finished the tea and the measurements she checked the size of my waist once more. "We'll have you looking your best," she said. "I love the pattern. You'll have to get six silver buttons the size of a threepenny bit and a nice square silver buckle. Goodness – look at the time. It's eleven o'clock. I'm off, I must get my beauty sleep."

Next day it was business as usual. When I sent for the new admission who had arrived the evening before, she waddled slowly into the room and I could see by her puffy eyelids that she had hardly slept.

As I examined her I asked if she had any idea when she was due. None of the girls knew how to calculate the date of their babies' births – I had to explain over and over how to add one week to the first day of their last monthly period and then add nine calendar months to that date.

She started to cry and poured out all her story to me. Her name was Mary. She was forty-four. She worked in Killarney, as a housemaid. Mary, just like Dympna at forty-three, imagined that pregnancy was impossible because of her age.

Soon she was getting morning sickness and went to the doctor to be told that she was pregnant. The man was scared that his wife would find out and Mary was too sick to continue her work as a servant so she went to a priest, a Father Billy. He arranged for her to come to the Home and promised to keep in touch. She was crying piteously at this stage and then she said, "God, Nurse, I was an awful fool. If he had no children with his wife, it was not his fault, anyway. What am I going to do?"

"If that Father Billy keeps in touch then you'll be luckier than most of the girls here as their parents have abandoned them," I said.

She was a very warm-hearted woman and after a few days, when she had settled as best she could, we became friends.

* * *

Julie, the little fifteen-year-old schoolgirl, was due in May and this was now March. She was very quiet and with her long hair down her back, she looked more like a twelve-year-old in the shapeless denim uniform and smock. It somehow did not seem right to see a mere child about to have a child. She got no special treatment from Sister. There were no favourites. They were all asked the same question over and over again:

"Was the five minutes' pleasure worth all this?"

* * *

The first fitting for my dinner-gown did not take place until well after eleven o'clock on the following Tuesday night. I had the six silver buttons and the silver buckle, but there was no sign of Sister Cyril. Sister was in the office and was also wondering what was keeping her. The dinner was on the following Friday night.

At ten past eleven, Sister Cyril came running along the

143

corridor with the frock on a hanger thrown over her arm, and her white ankles showing under her nightdress that was covered by the habit. She was out of breath and all apologies.

"Reverend Mother must be reading a novel," she said. "She has only now put out the light."

I took off my uniform frock and tried on the dinner-gown.

"It's lovely," she said. "It suits you. Have you no mirror here?" she asked Sister. "Never mind, turn around – it's perfect. Did you get the buttons and buckle? I have made the belt and put some canvas at the back and lined it in blue silk. The cape collar suits you and I don't think it's too low at the neck," she said, giving me a wink. It was low enough – just covering my cleavage! She was so different from her companion.

She asked if there was tea. We had no cake but we had some chocolate biscuits that night, and it was the bewitching hour of midnight before the two nuns left the office for the convent.

"I'll have the French Fern soap for you tomorrow, Sister," I called after her.

"You'd better," she said and was gone through the door.

Friday came and in the early afternoon, Sister brought over my ice-blue crepe dinner-gown on a wooden hanger. She took it up to my bedroom and laid it on the bed. I could hardly believe that this was the same nun who treated the girls with such indifference, and who could be and was very cross with me at times.

She enquired if I was ever at a dinner before?

"No. Only a dress dance and supper."

"This is totally different, Nurse," she said. "You'll have several courses and red and white wine. You drink white wine with fish and poultry and pork. Red wine with beef or lamb."

"I don't drink, Sister."

"Well, you may be offered a sherry before the meal." She then went on about *aperitifs* and *entrées* and *h'ors d'oeuvres* and so on. I was told at six o'clock that I could go off – she would do the bathing of the sixteen babies and supervise the breast-feeding.

I went off and had a hot bath and ordered just tea and toast at six as I was not sure what time I would be eating. I did my hair up in a French pleat and secured it with hair pins. I had borrowed a pair of diamante drop clip-on earrings from a friend of my mother's on one of my afternoons off. At last I slipped on the new blue gown and I felt good. There was no need for sun-tan lotion as the sleeves were long and I wore a light pink lipstick.

I was ready to be collected at half-seven at the hospital hall door. The usual four or five nuns were invited over by Sister and she told them who had made my frock. Sister Cyril beamed all over and I felt like Cinderella going to the ball. As was normal, I could hear the sound of footsteps as the girls rushed to the window to try and get a glimpse of us going off in the car. I felt so privileged when I compared myself to those poor desperate and desolate souls.

The night was magical. It was like nothing I was ever at before. The only hitch was a dentist who sat opposite me and asked where I was working.

"In a nursing home in Blackrock," I replied.

"Where is that? What name is it?" he asked.

"It's run by nuns," I said, blushing.

"Tell the man the name of the place," whispered Pat.

The dentist from Skibbereen said, "My wife had twins last year in the Glenvera. I never knew that there was a nursing home in Blackrock run by nuns."

I tried to change the subject.

The rest of the night went without incident and we ended up in the private house of the president of the dental association. It was three in the morning before we got back to the hospital. No light shone at the gable end, to my relief. At eight in the morning I had to face another day.

* * *

Easter was approaching and I was not sure if I would be allowed off for the two days. There was always this uncertainty about my time off. Christmas and Easter were not marked by any change in the monotonous routine – there was no hint of any celebration to mark either the birth of Christ or his Resurrection.

Pat was putting pressure on me to name the date of our wedding. At Christmas I had said that I would marry him in April. That month now seemed to be fast approaching and I once again said that I would definitely marry him in June as it was my birthday month, the reason for my name. On June first, my parents were celebrating their silver wedding anniversary, so I had to postpone my wedding once more until June 17th.

The week before Good Friday, I got a letter from my young twelve-year-old sister, saying she did not like Tralee and never ever got an Easter egg of her own. This was a pathetic letter so, on Spy Wednesday I cycled into the city and picked out a big milk-chocolate egg, complete with yellow Easter chick. It was presented in a box so I paid seventy-five shillings, and went to the bus depot to have it transported to Tralee. For this service I had to pay 3/6. Then in the fine drizzle, I cycled to the post office to send her a card to meet the bus the following day.

I then got the customary Green Door cake for Sister and cycled out to the Home, getting a fine wetting, as the April showers came with their usual furious frequency. I did not have time to have a hot bath before Sister called me to the office.

"Wait until I show you a photograph of Michael," she said.

"Who is Michael?" I asked.

"Last summer, an American lady called for a baby and she picked Michael, who was three. I'll read the letter for you." She was quite excited. It reminded me of the way she reacted when I was going to the dress dance.

The letter read:

Dear Sister,

I am enclosing a photograph of Michael and his nursery. He has settled in very well and my husband adores him. He met us both at the airport when I took Michael to the USA. He had a bouquet of white roses for me and a tiny bouquet of white rosebuds for Michael. We were a family at last!

Sister, you won't believe this but after fourteen years of marriage and no child I am now six months pregnant – it's a miracle. No matter how many children we may ever have, Michael will always be our firstborn.

Yours sincerely,

She did not read out the name. Sister then showed me coloured photographs of Michael and his parents – the garden, the swing, the house. His nursery had the smallest three-piece suite with a couch and two red leather armchairs. There was a rocking horse and toys and teddy bears.

"He is the lucky little boy," said Sister, as she folded the letter and returned it to the large envelope.

I wished that I knew where his birth mother had gone to. I felt as if I were being torn in all directions – glad that the little boy was being so well cared for, cross that the mother that bore and loved him for three long years had to let him go and then be cast out into a society that was uncaring and judgmental of her plight. I was glad that the woman in America was pregnant at last and yet so full of love for her adopted little boy. I felt ashamed that I had access to this information instead of the girl who needed it most. I felt guilty that I was afraid to voice my opinions of the rules here and most of all I wondered if I should be ashamed for questioning them in the first place.

"Nurse," she said. "You are drenched wet – why didn't you wear a scarf?"

I gave her the cake and said, "Give some to Sister Cyril." I knew I could not eat it now – the taste in my mouth was too bitter. I went up to my flat and changed into my uniform. There were babies who needed their bath and I needed to hold their warm soft bodies to make me feel real.

* * *

Later that night, my throat was very dry and I felt hot and cold. I went to bed early and prayed that no one would go into labour. I tipped that hatch above my bed and said a prayer – "Don't open tonight, please God". As if it was not far worse for the unfortunate girls that slept in the dormitory when their hour had come! There was hardly a night when getting into my bed I did not look at that hatch and hear the voice of the assistant matron in my training school: "No night duty – it will suit you down to the ground!' She forgot to tell me how difficult it was to get any nurse to work in the unmarried mothers' home.

I drifted off into an uneasy sleep until five when I awoke with a start. My mouth was like cardboard. When I tried to swallow, I realised that I had severe tonsillitis. With my head pounding and I shivering with cold, I did not need a thermometer to know that I had a fine high temperature. I struggled out of bed, got my dressing-gown from the wardrobe and put it on to stop the shivering. I waited until seven and when I heard one or two of the girls getting up. I opened the hatch and asked for Mary – the last woman that was admitted. I told her to tell Colette to tell Sister that I was not able to go on duty as I had a bad sore throat. She wanted to come into my bedroom.

"Don't come near me," I said. "You might pick it up. Sister can make her own decision as I have never been sick before. Just go to Colette, please Mary. She can tell the Sister after Mass."

I got back into bed and cursed the fact that I had got such a wetting on the day before. I was dozing uneasily on and off until Sister came up to my room to see for herself.

"Stay there," she said. "I'll send up tea."

"Sister," I said. "I couldn't swallow anything – my throat is so sore it's like swallowing broken glass." She took my hot-water bottle and said that she would send it up to me with a mouthwash.

I thanked her and cried into my pillow when she was gone. I was miserable and just prayed that I would be OK for Sunday when Pat came up to take me out. The girl who replaced Irene arrived up with a hot-water bottle and a glass of hot water and salt. She was different to Irene, and not as talkative.

At lunch time, Mary knocked on my bedroom door and came in, red-eyed. "Nurse," she said. "I am so sorry that you are sick. You remember Father Billy I was telling you about?"

I nodded.

"Well," she said. "He called up this morning from Killarney to see me and Sister came over to the convent to supervise the meeting. He told her that he had a position for me with a QC's wife in Chelsea after I have the baby. He wants us both to go over. Sister won't hear of it! Oh! God, Nurse – what will I do? He has it all arranged and she said that I must stay three years and won't listen to Father Billy."

"Mary," I whispered. "First you must have the baby – don't be upsetting yourself now. There's a good girl. We'll work something out. I hope you won't catch my sore throat."

"Is it true that you are leaving to get married? The girls in the dayroom told me. Jesus! What will this place be without you?"

I was using the mouthwash at the hand basin when Sister came into my bedroom. She had a half jar of iodine and a paint brush in her hand when she entered the room. It was a dark wet evening so she put on the overhead light.

"Is it any better?" she asked.

I could not say that it was. I just shook my head and felt my eyes filling up. The pain in my throat, especially when I tried to swallow my saliva was unbearable.

"Sit on the side of the bed," she said, " and here, put this towel around your neck." She took a pink towel from the rail by the hand-basin.

I opened my mouth. This reminded me of being nine years old with scarlet fever, when I spent six weeks in the fever hospital. Before I could gag on the brush, the searing pain when the Sister rubbed the iodine on my infected tonsil nearly made me cry out. The relief when she withdrew the brush was marvellous.

"I'll do that again in two hours time," she said. "Give me your hot-water bottle and I'll have it refilled for you. Get back into bed," she said and she disappeared out the door.

I held onto my throat. It all happened so quickly. I went back to finish the half-cold mouthwash – anything to get the vile taste of iodine out of my mouth. I was hanging over the hand-basin when suddenly there was a sort of a click in my right ear – as if something popped. Straight away there was pus pouring into my mouth and I spat it out under the running hot tap. The relief was immense and, as if by a miracle, the pain was going and soon the abscess was drained out.

I could swallow more easily now and got into bed in my dressing-gown and soon dropped off into a peaceful sleep. When I awoke it was dark and approaching nine o'clock. I could hear the stockinged feet of the ante-natal girls walking past my door.

Mary knocked and peeped in. "Sister is in the Surgery with a jar of iodine – I'm sure she's on her way up. How are you?" she said, keeping an eye out on the corridor for Sister's form.

"Much better, thank you, Mary. I'll see you tomorrow."

When she had left, I lay in the dark, thanking God

that the abscess had burst. I felt much better after the sleep. I was dozing again when the curt knock and the switch turned on announced Sister's arrival.

I sat up and said, "Thank you, Sister – my throat is much better. The abscess burst as soon as you went downstairs today."

"Are you sure?" she asked as she placed the jar and brush on the locker beside the bed. "I brought a flash lamp. Open your mouth." She looked at my throat. "Yes. It doesn't look so red and it's not as swollen either." She lowered the light to my neck. "What is that redness on your neck?" she asked.

"I put the hot-water bottle to my neck after the abscess burst."

"You seem to have an enlarged gland there now."

I assured her that I was feeling much better.

"I'll send you up tea and a few fingers of toast as you have not eaten all day."

I thanked her and she took the jar of iodine and brush away with her. I was hoping that I would have a letter from Pat in the morning. I did not know if I was to get up or stay in bed but Colette soon called in with the tea and toast.

"Sister said you were to stay in bed again in the morning." She sat with me while I ate the toast.

* * *

I got up after lunch the next day, Good Friday. I felt very groggy and the enlarged gland in my neck was painful but the soreness in my tonsil was better. I went downstairs and, only for the day nursery where the odd baby whimpered, the hospital was remarkably quiet.

I went to the kitchen, hoping to meet Sister Phillipa, but there was nobody around. I went to the dayroom but the door was open and there was not a girl in sight. I had never been in the hospital on a Friday afternoon as I usually was off to go to Mrs Crowe with forms or to the Dispensary in the village to register the newborn babies.

Normally the girls would be knitting in the dayroom but this particular afternoon the whole hospital was deserted except for the new mothers, around four of them, and one girl on duty with the new babies, giving Aspro bottles of sugar and water to any fretful baby.

Because of my bad septic throat, I did not want to go into the mothers' ward. By now, I was feeling very weak and there was cold perspiration on my forehead. I was just going up the stairs to my flat when one of the girls, Attracta, came up the corridor and stopped to enquire if I was all right. Sister had told them that I had a sore throat.

"Where is everybody?" I asked.

She blushed when she said, "it's the first Friday of the month, Nurse."

"Yes," I said. "So what?"

"The girls, all of us, have to go to the chapel to do a Holy Hour and we have to stand for a quarter of an hour, without moving, with our two arms outstretched." Her voice trailed off when she saw the expression on my face. "Please Nurse, don't say I told you. Sister says it is to make atonement for our sins."

I sat on a chair inside the dayroom. "Tell me, Attracta. Do the pregnant girls have to do this?"

"Yes," she said. "All of us. The convent girls have to put on their crochet caps and come to the chapel also from four to five."

I asked her if she was going to the kitchen as she had a Pyrex graduated measuring jug in her hand.

"I'm getting boiling water and sugar for two of the babies," she said.

I walked across to the big kitchen with her. The kettle was boiling on the Aga as usual. I got a jar of Nescafé from the press and took my cup off the already set tray and made a cup of coffee for myself.

"Would you like one?" I asked Attracta.

"I'd be afraid, Nurse," she said. "Sister might come over any minute. She told me to look in on the new mothers, too. Please don't say I told you about the monthly Holy Hour – a lot of the girls get weak." she said. "Like Mass – remember, Nurse, when you used to leave with one of us – you even came out with myself before I had the baby."

"Where is your baby now?"

"Over in the convent," she said. "I go over to breast-feed her but I work here in the day nursery. I'd better go," she said as she poured boiling water on a spoon of sugar in the jug. "Don't say I told you – I thought you knew, Nurse." She practically ran all the way back to the day babies' nursery.

I wearily wound my way up the stairs and sat in the sitting-room and wished that Pat would ring me as I could not make a call out. I only just hoped that the next day would pass and then it would be Easter Sunday and I would be away at three o'clock into another world.

The eerie silence of the hospital was finally broken by the sound of the sixty-odd waiting patients coming over the parquet floor of the corridor that joined the chapel from the hospital.

I could hardly believe that Sister, who showed such enthusiasm to me with the dances and dinners, could enforce such barbaric rituals on these poor girls.

SIXTEEN

JULIE IN THE GYM-FROCK

Saturday morning broke with a knock on the hatch above my bed. I was not completely over the sore throat, but there was no time to feel tired. I was quickly on my way to the dormitory. There I found Julie (who had come in in her Brigideen uniform) in an advanced state of labour. I reassured her that all would be well and left her to put on my uniform before helping her to get down the stairs to the labour ward.

Colette was still on night duty with Celine. Julie was very nervous and apprehensive, and I did all I could to reassure her that I would be with her all day. In the cold light of dawn, I felt very groggy but decided to get Julie into her gown and settled before I got a cup of hot sweet tea for her and myself. Sister would not be over to the hospital until after eight o'clock Mass.

I stayed with the girl and it was pathetic to see a mere

child of fifteen having the same excruciating labour pains as a married woman – nature did not change. I counted the time in between her contractions. They were coming now at ten-minute intervals – apparently she was getting a "show" all the previous day and the pains were coming through the night. I was told that the poor child knew that I had been laid up with a sore throat so she suffered in silence.

Julie was very reticent, as I remember. Perhaps her tender age made her so. At least she would not be doomed to spending three years there. At half-eight, Sister swished over in her white habit. She enquired how my throat was but said not a word about the poor child in advanced labour.

"Nurse," she said. "Will you manage here and I will supervise the bathing and feeding in the day nursery?"

I was glad to agree. She barely looked at Julie, whose face was contorted in pain, and left the room. I could see that everything was going to be as normal as labour could be. There was not a moan out of the girl. I had been told that between eighteen and twenty-four was the ideal time to have a first baby – I wondered.

They were so vulnerable and alone and without hope. This was the worst aspect of this place. It was all tears and toil and no help or hope and then the final amputation between mother and child, and the mothers never ever knowing where their beloved children went.

At exactly 10 o'clock on that Easter Saturday morning I saw that there was only a three-minute interval between the pains. I helped her onto her left side. "The next pain now, if you feel pressure, push." She did. This went on for fifteen minutes. Her long blonde hair was damp with perspiration. I was feeling very weak myself and hoped and prayed that Sister would not return from the nursery. The next ten minutes were the hardest. Julie squeezed my hand and muffled her cries and next thing I delivered a beautiful baby girl and cut the umbilical cord and placed her new baby daughter in the child mother's arms.

I could not help a tear of joy and sorrow as I waited for the afterbirth. The young mother cradled her baby in her arms as if it was the most precious gift. Sister walked into the labour ward.

"Why didn't you call me Nurse? You must be feeling quite weak."

Not a word to the newly-delivered mother. Sister had the £100 and the baby would go to God knows where. Julie would be free to go home in ten days after first breast-feeding her baby. I wondered if this was a form of economy or a cruel way of ensuring that the final parting would be more tortured?

Two girls helped me to carry her to the ward. I fixed her up and brought her tea and toast. I then returned to my flat for a cup of coffee in silence. I was so glad that it was I who delivered the youngest inmate during my stay at that place.

That afternoon, I just did the minimum as I was very weak after the quinsy and the enlarged gland in my neck was sore and tender. I longed for Sunday and Pat.

Mary was like a shadow. She was constantly waiting for me to tell me of Father Billy, who had all plans made for her escape. Sister still refused permission on the grounds that the baby might not be brought up a Catholic if they went to live in London. This seemed to be the priority – not Christianity as I saw it. But then who was I but a mere twenty-two-year-old? No words of mine could change the system there.

Sunday came and Pat was up on the dot of three to take me out to Mrs Long, his landlady, for Easter Sunday lamb and mint sauce dinner! She was better than a mother to us. My parents were in Tralee. Pat's father had died when he was a baby, and his mother died when he was eleven.

That particular Sunday, Pat drove us all to Innishannon after our lunch and Mr Long, her husband who was a train driver, showed us where he first "saw the light". We drove to the country church where he was baptised. The two men walked all around the church and Mrs Long and I visited the adjoining graveyard where there was a profusion of daffodils along a grass margin. We picked about twelve flowers each and we were admonished for "stealing from the dead" by Mr Long.

We explained that the flowers were not growing on anyone's grave. Mrs. Long said "Men are all the same". I felt as if I was in another country.

That night, Pat took me back to the hospital early as I was not yet fully recovered. The gland was still throbbing.

"You'd want to have that looked at," he said.

His concern made me want to cry and just stay in that car forever.

"I'm fine – just really tired."

He asked if I could try for a few hours off on Easter Monday as he could stay at his landlady's and call back to see me the next day.

This made me feel much better as I waved until the lights disappeared from view.

* * *

Easter Monday morning came very early for me. At six o'clock when Colette came into my room and told me a girl from Killarney (who worked as a waitress in a big hotel) was in advanced labour and was calling for me.

"I didn't want to put on the light in the toilet as we knew you had been sick."

I had been shot back to reality from a pleasant dream, and I wiped my half-opened eyes.

"Would you rather I call the Sister? I know how you must feel – you were very good to me when I had my teeth out."

"Colette, make me a cup of coffee and I'll be right down," I said. I fully realised that I had all the pluses and was privileged above all the misfortunates who were incarcerated in this sad place. I got into my freshly starched uniform and got a mouthwash before going to the labour ward.

The poor girl from Killarney was having a very difficult time. God love her, when she saw me she thought all her troubles were over. She was getting very strong contractions and had a bright red show – not a very reassuring sign. The foetal heart rate was going from 140 to 160 – very rapid.

I kept thinking of all the complications, like placenta praevia. Colette brought me the hot coffee. We adjourned to the ante-room.

"She is bleeding a lot. I wish the head would show," I said. "Do you think that Sister would ring for a doctor?"

"She never does," said Colette. "Remember the night

the girl had the dead baby – didn't you ask for a doctor then?"

I remembered. I will never forget the hourglass contraction that resulted in a stillbirth. In the next two hours, while the girls and Sister were at Mass, I encouraged the little waitress and rubbed her back which was causing her most distress during a contraction. Soon the head was showing and, after what seemed an eternity to me (what was it like for the unfortunate girl?) I delivered a nine-and-a-half-pound baby boy.

She was exhausted. She just lay there with her damp hair framing her pale face. I weighed the baby, wrapped him in a towel and tied the umbilical cord. We waited over half an hour for the afterbirth to come. The girl was shivering from cold, shock and loss of blood.

Colette had gone off duty. I was alone, the new baby was crying in the cot beside his mother. The afterbirth came and with it the haemorrhage started. It was like a torrent. I felt helpless. No amount of cotton wool would stem the flow. All I could do was an external massage of the fundus of the uterus. This is a most painful procedure but it was the only avenue open to me.

The poor girl cried out in agony and caught my wrist. I am ashamed to admit that I got cross with her and shouted *"Stop that – I must do this or you'll bleed to death!"* I was desperate.

"I'd be better off, Nurse," she said. "What have I to live for?"

Sister came into the labour ward and asked what was all the screaming about. That seemed to be biggest mortal sin in the place. The girl was exhausted. I was exhausted. The phone rang and Sister went up to the office to answer it and I had time to put my arm around the new mother and apologise for hurting her when she was having a post-partum haemorrhage. We both cried and I said "Look at your beautiful baby boy?"

She looked at him and stretched out her arms to hold him. The expression of love on her face wiped out the lines of pain and torment as she rubbed his cheek gently with her forefinger. After their special moment together, I took the big baby from her and placed him in his basket.

"His father was an important Englishman staying in the hotel, Nurse," she whispered. "And I was a fool."

I told her that I would get some tea and toast and whispered "I'm sorry" once more as I left the room. Before I could get as far as the kitchen Sister called me.

"Your boyfriend is on the phone for you, Nurse," she said. Her disapproval at the interruption was obvious. I was in no mood to apologise.

"I'm afraid," he said, "someone shot out of a side road and hit the front passenger door of the car last night."

"What?" I asked in shock. "Are you all right?"

"I'm fine, love. I'm trying to find an open garage but, as it's a holiday – I think I'd better go home. The boy who hit me said he'd fix the car as it was his fault. How are you? How's the throat?"

"I'm fine. I've just had the fright of my life with bleeding after a delivery."

"My God," he said. "You'll never stick that place. Will you please go to a doctor with that gland in your neck? I'm worried about you."

"I'm supposed to be the nurse," I said caustically.

"Some nurse – I wish you were out of there. I'll see you on Wednesday."

"I couldn't have asked for time off today anyway. We are very busy and I have a fifteen-year-old mother to help with breast-feeding today."

"I thought her child was being adopted on the tenth day?"

"So she is," I said. "They are the rules – look I must go, Sister is waiting for me."

"So am I," he said. "For all the good it is doing me."

Just to hear his voice on the phone helped to cheer my flagging spirits. I had really thought I had lost a mother that morning.

After lunch I spent a lot of time in the newly-delivered mother's ward, especially with Julie who was trying to breast-feed her baby girl. Suddenly, Sister came running down along the corridor.

"Get Nurse," I could hear her saying to one of the girls.

"There is a big complication," she said when I joined her in the office. "The schoolgirl's grandmother has died and naturally her father will wonder why she is not present at the funeral – her mother is frantic."

"Don't tell her, Sister," I said, meaning Julie.

"It's not her I'm thinking about," she said. "It's the excuse for her Father."

It amazed me that this nun, who was impervious to any of the girls' emotions or those of their mothers or sisters who admitted them was now, all of a sudden, looking for a valid excuse for the absence of the youngest of eight children from a funeral.

"The mother in Meath is ringing me back at half-four."

I sat down in the office. "Isn't her eldest daughter a Chemist in Dublin?"

"Yes."

"Couldn't her little sister have gone up to mind the children so that the eldest of the family could attend the funeral? Wouldn't that be a very likely situation?"

"Nurse, that is a great idea – I couldn't have thought of that on my own."

"There is no way the poor child could be present at the funeral with her new baby."

"I'll go over to the convent and ring her mother now and then she won't have to ring me later."

I went back to the mother's ward. The poor girl I had delivered that morning was sleeping peacefully and I put her new son out to the day nursery. "God love you, you need a blood transfusion," I thought. She was waxen. I warned the other girls not to wake her, and I explained that she had a very rough time.

I then went up to Julie who was smiling down at the bonny baby daughter in her arms, her long blonde hair falling down around her like a divided yellow curtain. I smiled at her and asked how she was.

"I'm fine, Nurse," she said.

"You're a great little girl at being a mammy at fifteen."

"I was sixteen a few days ago," she whispered.

As if that made any difference. She couldn't help letting a few tears brim over her beautiful blue eyes.

"What's up?"

"I wish I could keep her," she said as she hugged her angelic-looking daughter.

"I know – I wish you could too, but for your own mammy's sake you must go back to boarding school. Your daddy doesn't know anything and your mammy has paid £100 to Sister to find a good home for the baby."

"Will I never see her again?"

"Who knows?" was all I could say. "Give her to me now and I'll put her in the nursery. You go for a little nap because it will soon be feeding time again and you need your rest."

God love her; she kissed the sleeping baby and there were tears in my eyes as I turned and walked away to the nursery.

"Will I ever get used to the harsh stupid rules of this place?" I said to myself. I thought of all the harrowing cases I had met since I first came to work in this "no-night-duty wonderful" place. I thought of the poor frantic mother in Meath with her own mother dead and her youngest child, Julie, in a home with a baby herself. I thought of the £100 and how it altered Sister's conscience! I thought of my own privileged position in this house of despair and utter helplessness. I thought of my impending marriage . . .

My thoughts were rudely interrupted by poor Mary again waylaying me in the corridor. "Nurse," she said. "Am I due next week? Father Billy came up again today to meet me and to ask for my release. This is the third time I have had that poor priest drive all the way from Killarney and that bitch of a nun is positively rude to him. I don't know what to do."

"Come up to the surgery with me," I said.

As she lay on the labour-ward bed, I palpated her. I explained how the head is engaged three weeks before the birth date of a first pregnancy only.

"By God, Nurse," she said. "This is my first and my last."

"Yes, Mary," I said. "The baby's head is engaged in the pelvic brim so it's ready for the long or short journey. Dry

164

your eyes. I'm sure Father Billy will work something out. I never heard of any priest coming to anyone's aid in here since I came, so keep your fingers crossed."

She was one of the few who retained a sense of humour. As she heaved her bulky frame off the bed and tried to straighten the rough blue denim uniform and smock she said, "It's a pity I didn't keep my legs crossed, Nurse."

I could not help a smile. "I'll bet Father Billy will get you over to London yet. So cheer up."

"How is the girl from Killarney?"

"She is sleeping now," I said. "She had a son."

All that Monday, one episode followed another. Poor Mary was in tears and thought that the Sister in charge was telling me about Father Billy when she saw us in the office talking about the schoolgirl's problem of the grandmother's death. Sister never discussed any of the girls with me – except the Dublin girl, Marie, and her "silly mother" of forty and the schoolgirl's distraught mother.

After all the babies were settled for the night, I filled my hot-water bottle and had an early night. I kept waking that night – my mind was awash with the fear of losing a mother.

SEVENTEEN

MARY AND FATHER BILLY

The days were getting brighter and longer. The birds were singing every morning and the shrubs were a riot of colour. Daffodils sprung up all over the grass margins and in clusters under the willow trees. It was good to be alive but still the doom and gloom was palpable once inside the silent hospital. The noise in the kitchen and the cries of new babies were the only human sounds that filled either end of that long oak-floored hospital. Not even the muffled cries of the girls in labour could be heard outside the walls of the pristine labour ward.

It was on such a sunny spring morning that Sister opened out the two French doors that led onto a lawn full of bright green grass and a carpet of daisies.

"Come on, girls," she said. "Get down on your hands and knees and pluck the grass. Mind you pluck it sideways and don't pull up any earth. Put the plucked grass in your pocket – twelve on either side of the middle of the lawn and work backwards towards the high cement walls."

"Now," I thought as I folded the towels and spread some on the iron radiator to dry, "I have seen it all."

The poor girls looked a strange sight – one looking at the other to see if what they were doing was the right method. One girl from the convent came over with a wheelbarrow for the plucked grass and when it was full, she took it over to the compost heap on the farm.

I went down to the new mothers to help them with the breast-feeding and also to swab their poor torn perineums. It was only there I felt I was a nurse.

Sister never alluded to the grass-cutting to me, nor I to her. I was to see that operation many more times before I left. A beautiful manicured lawn with no implement used – only the hands of the pregnant and newly-delivered mothers.

One day she showed me a photograph of herself and her sister in the convent with the former Reverend Mother Rosamund and a familiar-looking Bishop. I asked who he was.

"That," she said with pride, "Is John Carmel Heenan, Cardinal of Westminster – he is our first cousin!"

I asked how they had the photograph taken.

"Oh!" she said. "He came and spent a weekend here and we could visit his room at night. On the Saturday, Reverend Mother took us out to Leopold's to have our photograph taken."

She was very proud of being a first cousin to a Cardinal and covered the framed picture very carefully in white tissue paper and put it in a press in her office.

* * *

It must have been about this time that I wrote to my father naming the date of our wedding. By return of post I got a letter and a cheque for £50 for my trousseau. I told Sister that we had set the date and that I was making my wedding cake with a Mrs Ryan, a neighbour of my parents before they went to Tralee, and a domestic economy teacher. Not long after Sister said one day, "Come over to the convent. The doctor is there and I'll get him to look at the gland in your neck."

My starched nurse's collar was rubbing against it and it was tender to touch. My sore throat was gone and I was feeling better – if a half-stone lighter! I went into the drawing-room of the convent and the doctor was standing on a hearth-rug in front of the usual empty, ornamental fireplace.

"I hear you are getting married?" he said as he looked at me.

"Yes," I said. "I am, doctor."

He looked at my neck and said, "You'd want to have that gland removed. You won't have much of a honeymoon with that."

Sister said nothing. I said less.

"When are you going?" he asked.

"I suppose the 3rd of June, I'll be leaving here . . . " my voice trailed off. I was so confused. There were only about six or seven weeks left of my time before I left. I thanked the doctor and wished to be excused.

That afternoon, the girl from Killarney waited outside the wash-room door for me. She had been been up a day or two and had a visitor over in the convent that afternoon. She handed me a box of Dairy Milk chocolates.

"There's no way I'm taking them," I said, "but thank

you just the same. Eat them all yourself – you could do with them."

"Please, Nurse – for all you did for me," she said.

I felt ashamed. Here she was, the poor girl who almost died, now facing three hard years. She tried to give me probably the only present she ever got for her baby, from another waitress who knew her story.

"Do as I say," I said. "Open the box and line your pockets and eat every one of them. Don't let Sister see them."

That afternoon, Mary told me "I have a bad back-ache and feel there is something going to happen."

"Don't worry – I'll be here and we will manage with Colette."

"Promise me," she said. "You won't call Sister over from the convent? I heard about the commode – the other girls told me. Can I call to your sitting-room tonight?"

"By all means," I said. "You know when Sister is gone to the convent the coast is clear."

During these last few weeks there had been several more admissions and the sorry sagas of the inmates seemed to be one continuous tale of woe with no hope. They all had very low self-esteem and all were filled with horror when they learned about their fate. In fact, in all the time I was there, the only one who stood out in my memory as being assertive was Marie, the army colonel's daughter from Dublin. She – God bless her – was a rebel.

As sure as night follows day, poor Mary went into labour the following afternoon and kept her labour pains to herself until Sister was safely settled in the convent. After an arduous labour she eventually was delivered of a lovely healthy baby girl before the April dawn. Colette and I were with her and she was exhausted when it was all over.

169

"No wonder they call it labour, Nurse," she said. "They forgot the 'hard'." She called her baby Frances.

Father Billy, true to his word had kept calling, kept being put off, and kept in touch with the QC's wife in Chelsea who promised a good home for Mary and Frances. Still the Nun would not sanction their release as the thought of them going to England seemed to bring with it the assumption that the child would not be brought up as a Catholic.

After a few weeks, Father Billy arrived up one afternoon with a wedding ring for Mary. Somehow – maybe Sister was in Shannon – he managed to get Mary and Frances away to the boat for England. The last words he said to her were "Remember you are a widow – your husband was killed in the Korean war."

I would never have known this except for a letter years later, and a snap of Frances on her First Communion Day in Chelsea. Mary wrote to me and said the lady she worked for had a cellar waiting when she arrived, all furnished with cot and playpen and high chair and go-car. Her own daughter had children of their own and all the baby things, including a dropside cot and clothes were in the basement flat for Mary and Frances.

And to jump ahead again, years later when I had four children of my own, my husband rang me one afternoon from his surgery in town to say that Mary had called with her little girl Frances and requested to see me. He told her where we lived and Mary's brother, a man of about sixty-five, drove her down to our house. We had tea in the garden and she told me how happy she was in Chelsea. Frances was going to a Catholic school in London.

"May God bless Father Billy," I said.

I never did hear his second name. But he stood by Mary and got her her freedom with Frances.

* * *

One morning, the new arrival to the surgery was a very tall thin woman from Waterford who told me that she was forty-seven. When I palpated her, I found the head in the fundus of her uterus (up under her ribs) and thought "My God, I'm in for trouble here, with the baby in the breech position."

I told Sister who showed the usual indifference – no question of calling in the gynaecologist. I just prayed that I would be able to deliver the baby alive. The woman went into labour around midday some days later, but as usual the other girls told her to wait until the Sister had gone off duty.

As I remember, she was a very quiet woman – not inclined to talk or pour out her history like the other much younger inmates. She hardly moaned during her labour. It was early morning. Again I had my faithful friend, Colette, who had witnessed hundreds of births more than I in her thirty-odd years. The baby's hind quarters were delivered. It was a boy. I knew the procedure on paper. I saw the long limp body of the baby boy and tried to insert my two fingers up into the baby's mouth and draw down the head by the chin to clear the pelvic brim.

I succeeded on the third attempt and I delivered the head of a six-pound baby boy, whose lusty cry was music to my ears! I was overjoyed – I had delivered my first breech alone and unassisted and the baby, though small, was healthy and strong. I placed him in his mother's arms and she kissed him.

"Thank you, Nurse," she said. "Isn't he beautiful?"

Mother love is universal and knows no bounds or barriers. I had witnessed it over and over in this place of misery and was always overwhelmed by the fact that the whole world seemed to be excluded during this one magical moment when a mother held her newborn infant for the first time.

* * *

It was extraordinary that the days that at first were so depressingly dreary were flying by, now that the final date of my wedding had been fixed. There was not another word about my sore gland. When the doctor had suggested surgery it was obvious that the idea did not appeal to Sister so it was never again mentioned.

Every afternoon I was off, there was the wedding and where we would live to discuss. All the flats and houses that Pat went to view either had no back yard or were not suitable for a surgery and dwelling house. Then there was the wedding list of relatives who were coming and those who were not coming if others were. One day Pat said, "I don't want to marry your entire family, only you – what is all the confusion about?"

But life went on much the same in the hospital. The admissions kept coming at a steady rate, and mothers and babies were sent over to the convent eight to twelve weeks after labour. Some were kept on until four months. These girls were useful around the hospital as the majority of the patients were innocent teenagers. Julie, the little school girl, went home with her mother on the tenth day. The final parting with her beautiful baby was a spectacle I did not witness, thank God. Sister never ever discussed where those babies went. I had realised since Dympna that she thought it was none of my business.

One afternoon when I was in the young mother's ward, Sister asked me to come to her office when I was ready.

"Nurse," she said. "Have you done anything about your Letter of Freedom?"

I must confess here and now that I did not realise that such a document existed. "Freedom from what?" I thought, I'm going to get married to a man I dearly love. I saw no problem.

Sister explained how the previous nurse got a Letter of Freedom from the priest and it cost her £20. I was aghast. Two months' salary? Where would I get that kind of money? My father's £50 was almost gone on my wedding dress and my going-away outfit.

"Nurse," she continued. "You'll need two letters – one from here and one from wherever you trained. If you are more than six months in a parish you need a Letter of Freedom."

I was stunned. Pat would not be up again until the following Sunday.

"You'll need to go to Confession to get a general absolution," she added for good measure. This, I thought, sounded easier and less expensive. But I was to find out to my cost that this was a bigger stumbling block!

It must have been the last week in April that I decided to go to Confession. I cycled into the city and entered a church where there were lights on over the confessional boxes. I looked around at the number of people waiting to go to Confession. If there was a queue it would be a sign that this priest was a nice or tolerant confessor. (How wrong I was!)

I walked up to the seat with six or seven people waiting to go to Confession. This seemed to be the most popular choice. I knelt at the outer edge and tried to examine my conscience. I had to make a General Confession. I racked my brain for major or mortal sins. The other people were coming out quickly – but they were not making a General Confession. I cursed Sister for trying to run my spiritual life. My mouth was dry, my heart pounded. I listened to the other penitents reciting the Act of Contrition and heard the *"absolvo te"* and suddenly it was my turn. The hatch flew open and I could see the priest. He was dark-haired and young – to me anyway – about thirty or thirty-five.

"Bless my Father for I have sinned, it's three months since my last Confession."

"What kept you so long?" he asked.

"I was busy – up at nights," my voice trailed off. "Oh! Father, I want to make a General Confession." I thought this would appease him.

"Why?" was the curt question.

"Because I am getting married in six weeks," I said with a certain amount of pride and relief. Now he can carry on from here, I thought to myself.

He asked me what I worked at that I was so busy not to have been able to come to Confession for twelve weeks. Actually it was more than twelve weeks and I then thought of the repercussions of telling a lie in Confession! I told him I was a nurse and then hoped that he would know that my workings hours were very irregular.

Then he said very solemnly, looking at me for the first time, "You know all about the marriage act?"

"Actually I don't, Father," I said. "You see, I have never been at a wedding."

He glared at me in the dim light of the Confessional and I could see the anger in his face and hear it in his voice. "Get out!" he said.

Just two words. I was stunned. I thought he meant the rites of the ceremony. As God is my judge, I did. I got up off my knees and went out of the box, bewildered as to what I had said wrong to draw his anger on me. I was out in the busy street with the watery sun of an April blinding the tears that came falling down my cheeks. I was absolutely shocked. I felt all the other people in the pew had heard him. I felt humiliated and cursed Sister for saying that I had to make a General Confession. What the hell did she know about it anyway?

My first thought was to cycle back to the hospital. Then I thought it would be another week before I would be off at six again. I pushed my bicycle up the crowded street. People were queuing for the pictures. I felt as if everyone knew of my dilemma and my rejection with a "get out" from the Confessional.

I had nobody to turn to. I could not ring anyone. I was confused and kept wondering what I had said wrong. It was not a sin surely not to have any idea of the ritual of the ceremony of marriage? I decided that I would try one more church and get it over with and not mention the General Confession. That seemed to have been my first mistake.

I turned off down a side street to a Franciscan church, and parked my bicycle. My eyes were blinded by the April sunshine until I was halfway up the side aisle of the dark church. Only the stained glass windows allowed any light in behind the altar. Up at the top, to the right of the altar, I saw the name Father Mel over the centre of one box.

I knelt and tried to gather my thoughts. I was more nervous this time but decided I would take a different approach. I looked up at the tabernacle and said to myself, "Please God, wish me luck". I am sure he had other more important things on His mind but just the same, I was doing my best.

When I finally got into the dark recess of the box, I heard once more the muffled voices on the other side. My heart beat faster. I thought of Frank O'Connor's "First Confession". This was far worse. I wondered if I knew the Act of Contrition. The hatch opened quietly this time and after what seemed like minutes the priest said, "Yes my child, can I help you?"

"Yes, Father," I whispered. "It has been twelve weeks since my last Confession." I tried to think of a few sins. Not that I was sinless, but usually I made up a few right-sounding sins like taking the Lord's name and losing my temper. I don't think I did much of either, but they sounded less innocuous than my own assortment. Then I blurted out I was getting married on June 17th. He turned around and looked straight at me.

"How old are you?"

"Twenty-three," I answered.

"What does your intended husband do?"

"He is a dentist."

"And what do you do?" he inquired.

"I am a nurse."

"Have you money?" he asked.

"No, Father," I said. "I am the eldest of six."

"Look, child," he said. "Dentists don't marry nurses. They and medical students have a good time with nurses, but they don't marry them."

I was getting cross. "I tell you, Father, I'm getting married on June 17th."

"Listen child," he said. "I am an old man. I know what I am talking about. Have you any idea how much it costs to set up a dental surgery?"

"My boyfriend is in practice for almost a year."

"His people must have money. Is he an only son?"

I explained that he was not. I had never met a confessor like this before.

"Listen," he said. "You are far too young at twenty-three to be getting married. You will have a rake of babies." [how right he was!] "Take an old man's advice, wait until you are about thirty or thirty-three and then get married."

I was really annoyed now and said with all the determination I could muster, "Isn't there such thing as the safe period?"

"There is," he said with a sigh, "but it doesn't work – you will have ten or twelve babies." He raised his right hand to give me absolution. After the usual Latin words he smiled and said, "The best of luck to you, God bless you".

I came out of there not crying, but not overly happy either, and I was slightly annoyed at the way he had said "Dentists don't marry nurses". I cycled back to the hospital and went up to my flat and wrote a letter to Pat. I was looking forward to going out with him on Sunday. I just needed reassurance that everything would be all right and decided there and then to go about my Letter of Freedom the next day, a Saturday, if things were quiet in the hospital.

EIGHTEEN

THE LETTERS OF FREEDOM

I decided to contact a Father Murphy O'Connor that I had nursed with a sore throat way back when I was a student nurse. Father Murphy O'Connor had come into one of the three private rooms in the hospital where I trained. At first, only the nun went into his room with the doctor and we students were confined to the public wards. Then after five days or so, the nun was put on night duty and I was asked to look after Father's tray as he was on light food now. I had to do scrambled egg on toast for his tea and set the tray properly.

The first time I saw him he offered me a cigarette which I declined, chocolates which I also declined, and asked me to sit down.

"We are not allowed," I answered.

"Goulding," he said, looking at my name badge. "Could you shave me?" he asked. "The Bishop is coming to visit me this evening."

"I'll try, Father," I said. I was used to watching my own father shaving with a brush and erasmic soap and a safety razor. I was naturally nervous and the procedure took about fifteen minutes. Father Murphy O'Connor was so pleased as he looked at himself in a hand mirror.

"Goulding," he said, "if ever I can do anything for you, you know where I am in the North Parish. God bless you, I feel better already!"

That was three full years before. I was wondering if he remembered me.

The following morning, after bathing the babies and examining about six pregnant girls in the labour ward, I went up to the office and requested to call Father Murphy O'Connor. Sister was agreeable. She was more worried about my Letters of Freedom than I was, so very soon I was talking to Father.

"I knew you wouldn't be long before being snapped up," he said warmly. "Of course, I'll leave it for you on the hallstand with my housekeeper as I'm going to the Canaries on my holiday this evening. It's a good job you rang this morning."

"How much do I owe you for that?" I asked.

"I never paid you for shaving me in 1948," he laughed. "Good luck," he said and was gone.

I went out and told Sister. I never told her the debacle with the two Confessions!

I had one more Letter of Freedom to get. The more I heard of the eighty-six-year-old Canon in the nearest village to the Home, the more I dreaded going up to visit him – especially as the nun kept telling me how the former nurse, who worked for seven years there, was charged the astronomical fee of £20.

It was nearly three weeks since my previous pay cheque and I had bought all the ingredients for my wedding cake as well as the almond icing. I was trying to work out a plan – I was determined to fight.

It was a wet Saturday evening and I had to go to Mrs Crowe with papers also. When I got to the back door, I passed two of the girls.

"Will you be long, nurse?" one of them whispered. "One of the girls has pains and a show."

"I'll be back soon – I never go out on Saturday nights so tell Carmel that I'll be back in less than an hour."

As I cycled up to the village, I checked in one of my pockets for the last green £1 note that I possessed before the next pay day. I said a prayer for Father Murphy O'Connor and I said several that my plan of campaign would work. I thought of the two Confessions with a certain amount of trepidation and the advice of the older priest rang in my ears.

Both my hands were glistening as I held on tightly to the handlebars with white knuckles.

"Oh! Please God, let it work," I prayed as I neared the bleak cement two-storied house. My heart was pounding as I pushed in the rusty gate and looked up at the dull, cream-coloured net window curtains.

I knocked on the rusty heavy iron knocker and waited. It was pouring steadily down and the leaking gutters were sending big heavy drops of rain along the front of the parochial house. After what seemed like ages to me, I heard the footsteps on the bare boards of the hall within.

The door was opened just a few inches to allow the housekeeper to peep out at me. I kept my hands in my pockets to produce an imaginary "bump" and kept my eyes down.

"What do you want?" she asked, not opening the door a fraction until she heard my request.

"I want the priest," I said, "or the Canon," I repeated.

"What for?" She eyed me from head to toe.

"I want a Letter of Freedom," I said, stepping from one side to the other to avoid the heavy shower.

She opened the hall door, exposing an equally dreary dark hall. "Come in, wipe your shoes and stand there," she said, slammed the front door and went up the hall.

I clutched my £1 and worried that my ruse would never work if he was as mad for money as Sister said he was. I am sure I looked a sad sight as I waited – I certainly felt it. I was so used to watching the pregnant girls waddle around the corridors of the hospital that I decided I might as well walk that way to make the "bump" look more authentic.

The door of the Canon's room opened and the housekeeper said, "Go in now, he'll see you." I waddled in and stood before a cluttered table. An old man in a greasy black suit peered over his glasses at me as I stood forlornly before him. The books and ledgers piled high on the table almost covered my "condition".

"Well, child," he asked. "What can I do for you?"

I told him that I needed a Letter of Freedom as I was getting married.

"What's your name?" he asked.

It sounded so incongruous to tell him my real name but a false one was no use on the Letter of Freedom.

"Where are you from?"

"Bessboro, Father."

"Oh! Good girl, you are doing the right thing." His gaze fastened on my mid-region over his glasses perched on the end of his nose. "When is the child due?"

I kept my hands in my pockets and said, "Soon, Father."

"Good girl. Himself? Where is he from?"

"The country," I said and he proceeded to write on a piece of paper, peering over the glasses every now and then at me. I kept my hand on the £1 and kept the "bump" out as far as I dared.

I could sense that the door was ajar and the housekeeper was listening to every word from outside. I was half-afraid that she would burst in any minute and ruin the whole thing. I waited. The clock on the wall ticked loudly and the April rain lashed against the window. Only the scratching sound of the nib on paper could be heard. He then handed me the paper – my prized Letter of Freedom. He got up off his chair and walked around to the door.

"You are doing the right thing," he said.

I was terrified. I turned and said, "Would you say Mass for me please, Father?" and handed him the hot £1 out of my pocket.

He grabbed it, saying, "To be sure I will, and good luck to you."

I waddled out into the rain and could hardly believe my luck. I had to go slowly. I felt the net curtains were being pulled aside to see the poor pregnant creature that was making an "honest" woman out of herself. I had to keep up the unnatural gait until I got around the corner and out of sight of the parish house. I was almost running to my wet bicycle, I was free.

I had made two General Confessions – one admittedly an abortive one. God bless Father Mel even though he told me to wait ten years, and God bless Father Murphy O'Connor. Now here I was cycling back on a wet Saturday evening to the hospital with my Letter of Freedom in my raincoat pocket.

* * *

I was in the hospital corridor by seven. All was quiet. Sister was over in the convent. I called two of the senior girls to enquire how Carmel was. She was getting pains, half an hour apart. I told her to hang on until after bathing time and then I would have twenty-four hours to devote to her before Pat arrived.

I had a hot bath and soaked all the April rain out of my feet, face and hair. I got dressed into my newly starched uniform and put my hair in a French pleat under the veil. In the nursery I showed Sister my second Letter of Freedom from the Canon and told her that he only asked for a £1 and promised to say Mass on June 17th for me – I did not elaborate! She was amazed at how little I had been charged.

At four in the morning Colette and I delivered Carmel of a lovely baby girl. I was so pleased with my day! I told Colette my story and we laughed in the warm kitchen as the Aga burned and another new baby was tucked up in the nursery for the night as a relieved eighteen-year-old country girl slept.

* * *

The following day was a warm April Sunday. Another patient had been admitted on the previous evening while I was at the village. She was forty-four and had been a Matron. The previous September, she went to Lisdoonvarna for the matchmaking week and had obviously got pregnant but not matched in marriage.

She had an elderly mother of eighty-four and two brothers who ran the family business. She was an only daughter and her aged mother did not know of her condition. Each sad story brought to this Home seemed to supersede the former in degrees of hopelessness. Apparently, the local family doctor, a 65-year-old widower, offered to marry her when he found out about her pregnancy. She declined.

Anne was her pseudonym, and she was a tall lady and nicely spoken. One could sense her embarrassment at being stripped of her lovely expensive woollen suit and camel coat when being admitted. She too, like all the other inmates, was divested of her undergarments – vest and brassiere and knickers. She too had to be humiliated by putting on the coarse denim dress and smock and the shorts with rough seams and a cord around the waist. Her bewilderment was obvious when Sister said, "Go with Nurse and she will examine you."

Now it was my turn to be embarrassed at the thought of palpating a woman of forty-four who had been a Matron or Ward Sister and was infinitely more competent than I! She had such a soft speaking voice, and beautifully manicured nails, too. One could see that she was certainly not the usual patient. She was very anxious to talk to me about her life and how she managed to get into this awful predicament.

I thought if Sister had pointed out the rules of this Home, she might have taken up the doctor on his humane offer. Already she was wondering what present she could give the kind Sister? She asked me about myself and how long I worked there. She seemed taken aback when I told her of my impending marriage in about six weeks. I was wearing Pat's beautiful engagement ring. I told the lady – as she truly was one – that I would not be here at the end of June or early July when her baby was due.

I kept thinking of her mother and the three hard years she would have to endure in this place, only to then part with her baby. I even suggested she contact the family doctor again. I did not see Sister treating her any differently to the other poor misfortunate abandoned girls. At this stage in spring the grass lawn in front of the hospital had to be plucked by the twenty-odd waiting girls every two weeks.

Anne was very talkative and it seemed to console her to chat to me when I was examining her and taking her blood pressure in the surgery. Her blood pressure was high and her ankles were swelling and I reported these symptoms to the Sister but my remarks were met with the usual callous indifference.

* * *

One Wednesday Pat was up before three. He was in great form. "I have solved the living accommodation," he said. "We have a flat out in the country for as long as we like and you can pick the house of your choice when we are married. All I want is to marry you and take you away

185

from this depressing place. Now it's time I bought you a wedding ring so you should try to get off on a Thursday or Monday morning in order to buy the most important gold ring of all! The date is set. My brother is coming to marry us and then the first thing we'll do after our honeymoon is have that gland in your neck investigated."

"There you go again," I said. "My throat, my cough, my gland, my head cold!"

"Well, someone has to look after you," he said. "You are very careless when it comes to minding yourself!"

I told him about Anne and how she had got pregnant in Lisdoonvarna after taking a few sherries. "It must have been great sherry," he said but stopped smirking when he saw my face.

I could not help telling him about the family doctor who offered to marry her. I thought anything was better than staying on here for three long years and then parting with her baby. I really felt very sorry for her. She seemed so very different and it was degrading to see her wearing the coarse uniform.

"Will you stop trying to take all their sufferings and tribulations on board? You are getting too involved here, and it's making you depressed and you should know now that you won't change the system or the rules. I'll meet you either next Thursday or Monday to buy the wedding ring. Ask Sister which day suits. Will you have all the twenty babies bathed by ten in the morning?"

"Shut up," I said. "You think this is all a big joke and I'm making up stories and that it's really a holiday camp and I'm just fantasising." I started to cry.

He put his arms around me and said, "The quicker I

take you out of here the better. Don't cry, June – I know you're upset to see so many poor abandoned girls. Count yourself lucky. I'm not abandoning you and you will soon be away from here and on my own property and all the past nine months will fade when you are my wife."

He could always cheer me up. I was just sorry in a way that I would not be around to deliver Anne. She seemed so totally out of place.

Sister put Anne sewing garments or uniforms with a hand-sewing machine. She had become more subdued. Sister was treating her as the other inmates – the morning rising at seven, the morning Mass, the frugal breakfast of milked tea and bread and margarine, the first Friday ritual of penance, the Saturday Confession with the chaplain, the silence, the rule against talking to each other or me . . .

I was embroidering in my sitting-room one lovely May afternoon, with my window raised up to see the beautiful flowering shrubs and to hear the blackbirds singing after the shower of soft summer rain, when one of the girls rushed up the stairs and stopped dead at the open door.

"Oh! Nurse, thank God you are there! Anne has got a sewing needle broken in her finger and Sister sent me up for you. She has got weak and is bleeding – come quick."

I dropped my embroidery and ran down to the sewing room. Poor Anne was slumped across the table with her middle left-hand fingernail punctured by the sewing needle. It had gone through her beautiful oval nail and the point was protruding in the middle of her finger pad. She had fainted.

"Can you remove the needle, Nurse?" said Sister.

"Would you open the glass case of instruments in the labour ward?"

Poor Anne was moaning and there was blood everywhere. I got an artery forceps and cotton wool and Dettol and a bandage and sticking plaster. One of the girls was with Anne, holding her around the shoulders.

I clipped the artery forceps on the broken sewing needle and held her wrist with my left hand. I pulled up and out came the needle and I elevated the arm to stem the bleeding and put on a dressing.

"Anne would need two Veganin for the pain and a cup of hot sweet tea for the shock," said Sister.

Poor Anne put her head on my shoulder and cried with relief. "Thank you, Nurse," she said. "Thank God you were here."

Sister walked out of the sewing room but before she did I told her that I thought that Anne should lie down for a few hours. Sister told one of the girls to clean up the mess, and another to replace the broken needle and to get on with the sewing. I helped Anne up to the dormitory and sat for a good while talking to her. I can still remember her asking me what present she should give to Sister, as her family or two brothers owned a big shop up in the midlands.

NINETEEN

LEAVING WITH A PROMISE

June 17th was fast approaching. Girls were still coming in and I was still doing most of the deliveries. I finally got a quiet morning off to buy the wedding ring, and Pat bought me beautiful earrings too.

Things were happening very quickly. Sister gave me an extra half-day one Tuesday when she heard that my Mother was travelling up from Tralee to go shopping with me. My heart was set on a red suit in Cash's, but I came out of the store with an oatmeal Glendale fashion fabric suit, a cream blouse and a flat pair of suede walking shoes as I was going to the country! To this day, I think of the red Barathea suit with the half-collar of velvet.

I was so totally disenchanted with my very ordinary oatmeal suit (to add to my dislike it had a brown vertical stripe!) that I did not show it to Sister when I returned, and instead hung it in my wardrobe with the cream blouse. I think it was the following morning as I was just after coming out from bathing the babies when Reverend

Mother Therese met me on the corridor. She was a most gracious English lady and spoke beautifully. She told me how sorry they were to be losing me. I was flattered. She then handed me a credit note for Dwyers in case I needed anything for the house or my trousseau, and told me to get what I needed.

I had read or heard that Princess Margaret had a grey flannel coat cut on princess lines and buttoned down the left side from a simple Peter Pan collar. I went in to Dwyers and got four yards of best light grey wool flannel and left it in to the tailoress with instructions. In this one thing, I did get my own way.

About two weeks before I left, I got an envelope from Mother Therese with a holy picture and a cheque for £25! When I showed it to Sister she said that the other nurse, who worked there for seven years, got a pair of Dripsey blankets when she left. I was astounded at Mother Therese's generosity.

I was getting letters from my sisters. There were wedding presents arriving to Pat and to my parents in Tralee. But things were just the same in the hospital. I was still looking after the new mothers and the deliveries, and there were still girls coming into my sitting-room at night on the way to bed in their stockinged feet. These few stolen moments of human contact, those special secret talks of their fears, hopes, desires, regrets – I could only listen. I knew in my heart that I could offer no solution for their awful predicament and worse still, no hope.

All I could give was a listening ear and a hug and a kiss on the cheek. I hope I gave solace to a few, but it was very cold comfort. Most of these nights, I went to sleep crying for those poor forgotten, forsaken and forlorn girls and crying with happiness at my own situation of being so near my wedding date.

Anne's bruised finger was very sore and tender. The needle surely punctuated the bone. Her lank hair and pallor showed up her age. The shapeless uniform did little to enhance her pathetic appearance. She was gone into herself – her lovely spontaneous friendliness had vanished with the dreary weeks of incarceration and her advancing pregnancy did little to lift her flagging spirit. I was sorry to be leaving as I thought she, above all, could do with a little kindness and I, again, wondered if she had ever regretted the gallant doctor's offer of marriage. If she had had any idea of the strict rules of this merciless Home, she might have had second thoughts.

Sister put her cutting out uniforms in the sewing room instead of sewing them. Her finger needed regular dressings – already her lovely nail had gone black and she had to keep it covered all the time. There was very little communication between us. I think Sister knew Anne had found a friend in me. This place was a plank that each girl had to walk alone.

Just before I left, I asked the Sister when Colette was getting fitted with her dentures. I pointed out, with my limited dental nursing care, that her stomach would suffer not having any upper or lower dentures. The Sister said she would have to wait twelve months to get them. I felt sure of my ground and knowledgeable enough to say that she could certainly get an upper denture at this stage.

Sister flushed with anger as she must have felt that I was "voicing an opinion" and I also had only barely two weeks left in the Home. My self-assertion amazed me, but I am afraid that it was too little, too late.

* * *

One beautiful Wednesday afternoon in May, I was
waiting in my sitting-room to be collected by Pat. I had
started to pack some of my handmade trousseau and
embroidered cloths and tray cloths. I was dressed in a
pink linen polka-dot summer suit and my hair was
pinned up in a French pleat – I missed Maureen's bi-
weekly hair wash and set. I often wondered how she was
getting on in Moorepark. Her baby had been sent out to
St Finbarr's Hospital for possible cardiac surgery.
Maureen's mother wrote once, with a beautiful hand-
knitted cardigan for me for the only small kindness I was
ever allowed to show to her daughter.

I caught the pungent odour of fresh tar, wafting its
way up and through the muslin curtains that hung on my
bedroom window. I thought at last the road workers had
come to fill in the many potholes on the long curving
avenue that led from the black wrought-iron gates to the
hospital and over beyond the rhododendrons to the
nuns' convent. I often almost went into some on my
bicycle – no wonder I loved to be driven on a Sunday and
Wednesday. I was busy packing and tidying drawers when
I heard the familiar sound of Pat's black Prefect – only a
couple of weeks to go!

I got my handbag, and slipped on my white sandals
and ran down the oak corridor and down the staircase
past the dayroom door. I could hear the pregnant girls
saying the rosary out loud as they knitted.

Pat was wearing a lovely new beige sports coat and a
green shirt.

"Now I have seen it all," he said, as I got into the car.

"What do you mean?" I said, the smell of tar permeating the air now to a nauseating degree.

"Close your window," he said. "But keep your eyes open."

As he turned the car and eased it down the avenue, we rounded a clump of flowering shrubs. Then I saw them, about eight to ten girls, all in varying degrees of pregnancy, with heaps of gravel, a fire burning to heat a black bucket of tar and a roller that took three pregnant girls to pull. Pat drove in first gear and stopped when one tall girl came up to his window.

"Mind your tyres, sir," she said. "Go around on the grass – we'll have the whole avenue done before you bring Nurse back to-night."

"Thank you," was all he could say.

The other girls waved at me on my side of the car as Pat took a deep swing into the thick green grass that was on either side of the tarred avenue.

"I think that is the worst sight I have ever beheld," he said when he got out on the road. "You told me about conditions in there, about the plucking of the grass, the cross-cut sawing of the timber, the ploughing and the conditions of life behind those high cement walls, but I never imagined it would feel so terrible to see for myself."

I was looking at him, wondering if he had thought I had made it all up.

"I thought you were exaggerating, but this tarring episode is the last straw. How long more do you have in there?" he asked as we sped away on the road to the city. "Today I am going to take you to the sea – it's such a warm May day and you'll get the smell of the tar and that

193

hospital out of your lungs. We'll go to a show to-night. I hope that none of those girls will go into labour after the heavy manual work – God! What kind of a creature is that nun who runs the place? You told me about some of the harsh rules in the hospital, but to have pregnant girls doing that heavy manual labour is not right."

I think this was the first time that Pat became fully aware of what I had been trying to explain to him. He could hardly believe his own eyes. All evening he kept alluding to the avenue and the way the tall girl had promised that it would be finished by tonight.

"It's incredible," he said. "Men make their living tarring roads – have these girls no rights?"

I was weary and upset that this spectacle had almost ruined an idyllic afternoon by the sea. I knew where I was going to live after my marriage was very far from the sea. As we walked hand in hand across the golden sand of the deserted beach, I just wished that Pat could forget what he saw. He could not change the rules there either.

"They have no rights," I said. "Once they enter the gates they lose all rights about themselves, their bodies, their souls, and also all rights to their babies or their whereabouts. I have spent nine months there and now all I want is to be free because in a way I am also a prisoner. I cannot voice my opinions and I know whenever I tried I was shot down. Nobody nor nothing will change the regime in that place." I then reminded Pat that he thought I would never be out of my first private nursing case.

"Yes, I was afraid for your health and now you have an enlarged neck gland due to a neglected streptococcal throat."

"Anyone would think you were a doctor the way you carry on," I said.

"Anyone would think you were a nurse and a midwife also!" he said with a laugh as he stomped at the water's edge to splash me.

On the way to a hotel for our supper, we talked about our wedding. I said, "My best friend, who met me in Dublin with the baby for the Home in Blackrock, will be coming. Apart from my parents, one uncle, one aunt, my two younger brothers and three younger sisters, that's the sum total of the guests bar my mother's friends!"

"Whose wedding is it? Your mother's or yours?" he asked and I felt like agreeing with him.

After the Opera House, we drove back to the hospital. The moon shone on the newly-tarred winding avenue. The odour of tar was not as pungent in the cool night air. I closed my eyes. I was so completely happy and content, after a wonderful afternoon and night. Pat looked up at the familiar beacon in the top of the gable of the hospital.

"Don't open your eyes, sweetheart," he said. "Keep them closed, think of this afternoon, the sea and the sand. I hate to interrupt your reverie but there is a light on, telling you that your skills are needed."

I sat up and saw for myself. I tried to recollect who was next on the delivery list. Pat stopped the car at the back door.

Colette ran out. "I'm sorry, Nurse, one of the girls is nearly ready to be delivered. I was just going to ring Sister but she begged me not to and then I saw the lights of the car."

"I'll be off then," said Pat.

I flew into the labour ward. The baby's head was showing. I had barely time to put on the red rubber apron and scrub up and put on the rubber gloves. Another baby entered the world. I asked if his mother had been on the avenue that afternoon.

"I put the shovels of gravel on the hot tar, Nurse," she said as she cuddled and kissed her son.

Once we had settled them both, I retired to the kitchen with Colette with our tea and hot buttered toast. Poor Colette held her hand over her edentulous mouth for most of the time that she was talking. I told her that I had suggested to Sister that she got at least an upper denture to help her to masticate her food. She was grateful. I could see that she was all apologies for calling me in from my date.

"Don't worry, Colette," I said. "We had a lovely afternoon by the sea. Seeing the girls tarring the avenue really upset Pat this evening."

"I remember doing that before I had my son. That goes on every summer, Nurse," she said.

I met Anne, the next morning, as I was about to go up to my sitting-room to write a letter to Pat. Her finger was very sore and she told me that she was awake a lot of the night as it was throbbing. She was crying. She looked utterly dejected in her uniform. I turned back. A letter could wait.

I took her to the surgery and opened the dressing. Her nail was black and the finger was swollen – it was infected. She looked at me and I tried not to meet her gaze. We both knew that she should be on antibiotics.

"I'll get a bowl of hot water from the kitchen and I have boric lint in the surgery," I said.

We bathed the injured finger for ages and she told me more of her family situation. She had worked in England for most of her life. The Lisdoonvarna affair was very puzzling to me. I did not know if the family doctor had taken her there and had taken advantage of her or if he offered to marry her when he found out about her condition.

She was very confused and I wondered if Sister had promised to have her baby sent to America for the £100 fee. Once inside the institution there was no way out – at least that's what the poor unfortunate inmates thought. They were as free as the wind – provided that they had a safe haven to go to, but where? In a country town, it could not have been a bigger scandal, particularly for a 44-year-old Matron.

I tried to console her and asked if the doctor's offer was still open. She assured me that it was and that he was a kind man and a family friend, but that Sister advised her against this move as she would get the baby to America for £100. At this stage, Anne could not associate a baby with the cumbersome bump she was carrying about. The tears of despair and pain coursed down her ashen face. I wish I had it in my power to ring that doctor to come and rescue her and take her from this godforsaken place. Again I felt helpless.

"Nurse," she said. "The abscess has burst – the hot water has done the trick, it feels better already. It's a bit numb but all the pain has gone. I feel a bit better after talking. For your age, you are wiser than I."

"Not wise, Anne," I said. "Lucky." I put a fresh dressing on her finger and slipped her two Anadins of my own.

"It's a pity you are leaving – what should I give Sister for a present?"

"Wait until you have had your baby."

I never knew what happened to Anne or what became of her baby, boy or girl. Except for Mary, who went to Chelsea with Frances, I never kept in touch with any of the girls.

But in 1990 I got a telephone call from a "Sheila" with a strong Northern English accent.

"Don't you remember me?" she asked on the phone.

"I can't say that I do," I said.

"Don't you remember 'Molly' in 1951? You got me to go to Huddersfield."

"Oh! God, Molly! I often wondered where you went! I heard you had got married."

"Well," she said. "I am in the Blarney Hotel now with my granddaughter who is eighteen – she is Patricia's eldest."

We met. We talked. We cried. She is still in constant contact with me and is the only one who can verify that the story I have told is the truth. In fact Sheila can say that it was even more horrific to find oneself at twenty, pregnant by a boy who died of tuberculosis, and cast away to a place that made the fear and pain go on and on.

I am digressing. This saga is nearing completion. My wedding was getting closer and Sister handed me a white cardboard box, with a blue rosary beads inside, one day. Sister Cyril wanted to knit a bed-jacket for me but Sister did not encourage me to buy the wool for her. I thanked her and reminded her of the lovely dinner-gown.

I had decided to leave two weeks before I got married, on June 3rd. I knew I would miss all those girls terribly even though I was leaving to marry the man I loved so dearly.

* * *

I awoke at the dawn on June 3rd, 1952, to a beautiful bright cloudless sky. I turned to the muslin curtains and thought – today I am leaving. The night before I had said a tearful goodbye to Colette.

I got up and dressed and went to Mass for the last time. I knelt at the back of the small church and saw the crocheted caps of the three hundred odd girls that inhabited the Home. I tried to concentrate on the Mass. My thoughts were many and varied, and my memories kept crowding in – the first enthusiastic days of "no night duty" and then the appalling reality that this was not a hospital or a home, but a place of detention for the poor creatures who found themselves bound to stay here for three long tragic years.

I thought of all the rules and the humiliations that the inmates had to undergo. I was not very proud of my stewardship. I could do nothing to alleviate any of the suffering of any of the girls. Molly was my only achievement.

I went to my breakfast in my bedroom. There was a pile of newly laundered nurses' dresses, calico aprons, collars and veils on my bed. The girl in charge of my meals had brought up the breakfast. I thought of Irene and her little son Seán, who went away, where she never knew. Where was she now? Where was he?

I ate the smallest breakfast as I was naturally upset at leaving and still wishing that I could have done more to change the archaic rules of the Home. I was glad that I had helped Dympna. I had no regrets that I ha' contacted her sister and helped to secure her freedom

I had no regret that I had helped Molly and Patri go to Huddersfield to work for Vincent, my brother-in-law. I let Sister know that I disapproved of keeping a girl on a chromiur practically for the entire labour. I also disapproval when Sister told poor mental' to get dressed and go back and fin' corridor. These, and a few more inc'

.y memory of working as a midwife in such a joyless place where even the birth of the Infant Jesus at Christmas was not recognised.

I had to spend all day on duty as Pat was working and would not be up until eight o'clock to collect me and my few belongings. I watched the girls being sent out to pluck the grass. I was hoping that Anne would not be included, but as I might have guessed, when I looked out the window she was among the twenty girls who were on their hands and knees.

I went out to the lawn, strewn with daisies in the warm June sun. I called Anne. She levered her cumbersome body into an upright position.

"I need to check your blood pressure," I said.

The other girls worked on. Anne had her finger bandaged and the tears were brimming over in her sad dull eyes.

"Come with me to the surgery," I said. "I need to dress that finger."

"Are you leaving today?" she asked.

"Yes, later this evening."

I dressed her finger and took her blood pressure. It was high. She looked at me and I could not help asking if she was right in turning down the offer of marriage. She said again that Sister promised to get the baby a place in America when it was born, for £100. There was no use in arguing with her. Obviously Sister had been in touch with some childless Americans.

I advised Anne to go to the sewing room to cut out tterns as Sister was over in the convent that morning erviewing some American people who had come to pick the few babies who were chosen to put be on display, essed up and looking wide-eyed at these strangers.